The Transplant Imaginary

The Transplant Imaginary

Mechanical Hearts, Animal Parts, and Moral Thinking in Highly Experimental Science

LESLEY A. SHARP

UNIVERSITY OF CALIFORNIA PRESS

Berkeley Los Angeles London

University of California Press, one of the most
distinguished university presses in the United
States, enriches lives around the world by
advancing scholarship in the humanities, social
sciences, and natural sciences. Its activities are
supported by the UC Press Foundation and by
philanthropic contributions from individuals and
institutions. For more information, visit www
.ucpress.edu.

University of California Press
Berkeley and Los Angeles, California

University of California Press, Ltd.
London, England

Library of Congress Cataloging-in-Publication Data

Sharp, Lesley Alexandra.
    The transplant imaginary : mechanical hearts,
animal parts, and moral thinking in highly
experimental science / Lesley A. Sharp.
        pages   cm
    Includes bibliographical references and index.
    ISBN 978-0-520-27796-0 (hardback)
    ISBN 978-0-520-27798-4 (paper)
    1. Transplantation of organs, tissues, etc.—Social
aspects—United States.   2. Ethnology—United
States.   3. Medical anthropology—United States.
I. Title.
    RD120.7.S492   2013
    174.2'97954—dc23   2013024442

Manufactured in the United States of America

23   22   21   20   19   18   17   16   15   14
10 9 8 7 6 5 4 3 2 1

In keeping with a commitment to support
environmentally responsible and sustainable
printing practices, UC Press has printed this book
on Natures Natural, a fiber that contains 30%
post-consumer waste and meets the minimum
requirements of ANSI/NISO Z39.48-1992 (R 1997)
(Permanence of Paper).

For my father
Rodman Alton Sharp
D.O.D.
1930—2013
A man who found beauty both in nature and in the tinkerer's art

CONTENTS

ILLUSTRATIONS

As an anthropologist and ethnographer, I am extraordinarily dependent on—and deeply grateful to—the many people who have so willingly and graciously given of their time throughout the course of this project. Ethnographic research often approximates a remarkable journey through uncharted terrains of human experience and, inevitably, the self. Given that this project has spanned over a decade of research, the task of recognizing and thanking all who made this work possible, intriguing, and rewarding is inevitably impossible. Here I offer a feeble attempt to recognize those who have assisted me along the way.

To begin, my research simply would not have been possible without the generous, sustained financial support from a range of sources. A summer residency in 2002 as a North American Visiting Scholar at the Hastings Center for Bioethics in Garrison, N.Y., formally marked the onset of this project; there, I mined the small yet impressive archival collection on xenotransplantation and had numerous discussions with the seasoned staff bioethicists, whose ideas specifically about the scientific use of animals profoundly shaped my own thinking. I remain to this day deeply indebted to them, especially for the fact that they never treated my questions as misguided or quirky. A post in the summer of 2006 as an Ethel-Jane Westfeldt Bunting Summer Resident Scholar at the magnificent and friendly retreat of the School for American Research (now the School for Advanced Research) in Santa Fe, N. Mex., hosted both me and my family and enabled me to draft subsequently successful research grants that would support this project for the next four years. I am especially indebted to Nancy Owen Lewis and James Brooks for their warm encouragement and ongoing interest in my work. I will also be forever grateful to Michael Banner of Trinity College, University of Cambridge, in the United Kingdom, who has sponsored not one but three separate events that have facilitated my research in deeply inspiring ways, coupled with a summer residency there in 2010, again with my family in tow. His influence has been especially profound in terms of reshaping my thinking about the intersection where moral philosophy, bioethics, and anthropology converge.

Barnard College, in turn, has been wonderfully generous and supportive throughout, providing a range of funds that reflect the college's ever-expanding vision and ability to think across disciplinary boundaries. These include a Mellon Foundation Seven Colleges New Directions Fellowship in 2003; a departmental grant through the Kraus Fund (2008-9); an Environmental Sciences grant, paired with a Faculty Mini Grant, which together enabled me to probe the moral pitfalls and interspecies dangers associated with animal research (2007-9); and a Translation Grant (2009-10), which, with Peter Connor's support from the French Department, funded exploratory work on the burgeoning field of "translational research" in medical science. These internal funds also provided seed money that enabled me to generate the data necessary for applying for larger outside funds, first from the Wenner-Gren Foundation for Anthropological Research spanning 2003 to 2005 (Grant #7010) and subsequently the National Science Foundation from 2008 to 2011 (Award #0750897). (Any opinions, findings, and conclusions or recommendations expressed in this material are mine and do not necessarily reflect the views of the NSF or other institutions.) I am especially indebted to Deborah Winslow, who encouraged me from the start to apply for NSF funding when I made an initial inquiry years ago. Invaluable support for a year's uninterrupted writing was provided by a Tow Family Award and a Presidential Research Award, both through Barnard College. In turn, gifted, patient archivists based at the University of Utah, Tulane University, the University of Michigan Medical Center, Columbia University, and the Rockfeller Archive Center, Sleepy Holly, N.Y.; artists Tim Wainwright and John Wynne and Fiber Artists @ Loose Ends; media experts at Syncardia Systems, Inc., Thoratec Corporation, and the University of Arizona Medical

Center; and staff at the Smithsonian Museum and the Eli Whitney Museum at Yale University all proved to be remarkable sleuths in assisting my efforts to track down documents and images. Thank you, all.

Many others, too, have provided support in a range of ways. I am deeply thankful to my father, Rodman Sharp, who died just as I was completing this manuscript. As a nuclear chemist, inventor, and investor, he understood from the start the relevance and timeliness of this project. My son, Alex Fox, who shares his grandfather's fascination for seemingly impossible hybrid configurations, has long provided much inspiration, not to mention lots of love and wicked humor (sometimes with a little help from the adorable Zookie). I thank Andy for accompanying me and Alex on research jaunts and for sometimes holding down the home front during my travels. May he find sustained joy in his future travels. My brother, Erik Sharp, has inevitably provided whimsy and thoughtful critique throughout. Others who have sustained me include Ruthie and the late, beloved Wally Kreisman, the late Mary Bradstock and Frank Bradstock, Erika Doss, Vanessa Uelman, Lisa Tiersten, Tovah Klein, the Tuttles, Emily Zants, Susie Blalock, Steve Foster, Louis Dorsy, Lucy Painter, Malaga Baldi, Heather Altfeld, Paula Rubel, Abe Rosman, and Maxine Weisgrau, alongside the gifted talents of both J. Beldner and R. Carmen. Good cheer, loving support, and pithy comments from all on the sometimes absurd nature of what I do have proved invaluable. I have drawn inspiration over the years as well from my wonderful colleagues and students in Anthropology and elsewhere at Barnard and in Sociomedical Sciences at Columbia, most notably Nadia Abu El-Haj, Sev Fowles, Stephen Scott, Paige West, Liz Boylan, Linda Bell, Jennifer Hirsch, Kim Hopper, Richard Parker, Carole Vance, Chris Alley, Emily Cohen, Kirk Fiereck, Robert Frey, Brendan Hart, Gina Jae, Laura Murray, Will Voinot-Baron, and Nancy Worthington, and from such dear colleagues as Nancy Chen, Peta Cook, Faye Ginsberg, Linda Green, Sarah Franklin, Stan Holwitz, Klaus Høyer, Marcia Inhorn, Anja Jensen, Sue and Simon Kenyon, Katie Kilroy-Marac, Shirley Lindenbaum, Julie Livingston, Margaret Lock, Monica Mann, Emily Martin, Mary Beth Mills, Lynn Morgan, Gísli Pálsson, Rayna Rapp, Carolyn Rouse, Rhonda Shaw, Marilyn Strathern, Zoe Strother, Mette Nordahl Svendsen, Janelle Taylor, and Jen Van Tiem. I could not have hoped for a more talented crew of research assistants: Ann Brink, Sumaiya Khalique,

Daniele Lerner, Sonya Rubin, and Chomee Yu were experts in every way imaginable. Special thanks to Jessica Goldstein for teaching me how to dissect a fetal pig. And many, many thanks to the gifted editor Naomi Schneider for her enthusiasm and support for this project from the very start. Kudos as well to Press staff who oversaw in expert fashion the production of this work, most notably Chris Lura, Jessica Moll, Lia Tjandra, and Julia Zafferano.

Finally, I am forever indebted to the many scientists who gave of their time, tolerated my questions, and showed interest in my research, not to mention the quirky nature of anthropological probing. Out of respect for their privacy, I refrain from identifying them by name. I will, however, make one exception: it is difficult to describe the level of inspiration I have derived from Peer Portner, a nuclear physicist, bioengineer, and pioneer in the field of VAD design who died at the age of 69 in 2009. The depth of his ethical thinking about the nature of his own field was truly exceptional. Among my most pronounced regrets is that I did not have the opportunity to befriend him for a longer period of time. I also wish to thank by name Peter Houghton (1938–2007), whose life story touched me deeply. He should be an inspiration to us all.

Introduction

Moral Neutrality in Experimental Science

On August 2, 2011, the BBC reported the successful hospital discharge and homecoming of forty-year-old "dad Matthew Green," who had undergone an extraordinary surgical procedure two months before: a team of transplant experts permanently removed Green's failing natal heart and replaced it with a SynCardia Total Artificial Heart (TAH), a device designed to serve as a temporary "bridge" until a suitable human donor heart match could be found. Green's newly implanted artificial heart was now powered by an external Freedom® Portable Driver,[1] a hefty battery assemblage weighing a bit over six kilograms, or thirteen pounds, tethered to Green's body and nestled within a backpack that he must carry at all times. Reports of Green's story played on long-established tropes that emphasize both medical prowess and regained social normalcy that were first developed two decades ago by the U.S. transplant industry and have since gone global. Green's case is one of approximately 900 similar surgeries worldwide, although his marked the first attempt in the United Kingdom. As cardiovascular surgeon Steven Tsui proclaimed, this was "the first time a patient was walking the streets of Britain without a human heart."[2] Green himself underscored the effects of his surgical transformation in words reminiscent of those uttered by recipients of allografts (that is, transplanted organs derived from human donors); as he explained, "It's going to revolutionise my life. Before I couldn't walk anywhere. I could hardly climb a flight of stairs and now I've been up and I've been walking out and getting back to a normal life. . . . I went out for a pub lunch over the weekend and that just felt fantastic, to be with normal people again."[3]

The simultaneous celebratory tone, themes of urgency and miraculousness, and a matter-of-fact approach encountered in Green's story typify accounts of mechanical hearts and other highly experimental forms of nonhuman organ replacement. Involved professionals regularly underscore chronic organ scarcity as legitimating highly experimental transplant procedures, an approach that is paired with triumphant proclamations of scientific ingenuity. For instance, Green's surgeon, Tsui, has consistently featured the TAH as a crucial life-saving technique in a hospital that performs over 2,000 heart surgeries a year yet is plagued by a chronic shortage of transplantable hearts. As explained by Peter Weissberg, medical director of the British Heart Foundation, transplantation may be the "only hope of long-term survival, but donor hearts are not always available" (BBC 1999). The TAH thus stands out as an important example of medical prowess, as exemplified in the words of Health Secretary Andrew Lansley, who responded to news of Green's story by declaring that "The NHS [National Health Service] has a long and proud track record of innovation that has driven major improvements in patient care in the past" (BBC 1999).

Green's TAH has, unquestionably, extended and temporarily improved his life. Oddly, though, no detailed account exists to date of the suffering Green endured as the subject of an experiment that necessitated the permanent removal of an organ many equate with vitality, love, and life itself. Green unquestionably endured an arduous, highly invasive, and life-threatening surgical procedure, one followed by two months of hospitalized recovery. One need only consider the history of Green's TAH to uncover potential pitfalls, because his implant is an advanced version of the Jarvik-7 device, its precursor implanted decades before in Barney Clark, a sixty-one-year-old retired dentist remembered as a "pioneer patient" in artificial heart design, a man who underwent surgery at the University of Utah and who survived 112 days while tethered to a power driver the size of a washing machine. As others subsequently reported, for instance, "Clark's implant robbed him of his freedom, binding him to his bed and causing constant infections and several strokes."[4] Although the cumbersome and clunky nature of the Jarvik-7 is in many ways a far cry from the contemporary SynCardia TAH with its portable backpack, Clark's early experiences nevertheless help raise vital questions in a context where surgical survival and postoperative recovery expose a mystifying black box of medical intent and care. How might we encourage questions about physical and psychic suffering endured by patients like Green? What of the private sentiments of a man whose heart is now artificial and powered by a hefty external driver? How do family members, friends, acquaintances, and strangers respond to someone who has no heartbeat and whose body must now sport opaque driveline housings protruding ostentatiously from his abdomen?

These are the very sorts of questions that drive *The Transplant Imaginary*. At the heart of this work, so to speak, are deep concerns about the inevitable yet silenced nature of patient suffering, paired with professional sentiments about the urgent necessity and celebratory qualities assigned to scientific inventiveness. This experimental ethos has long defined the very core of human-to-human organ transfer (also known as allotransplantation), and associated sentiments likewise now pervade a range of alternative and highly experimental forms of human organ replacement. As I detail below, alongside TAH technology one encounters the competitive domain of xenotransplant research, where involved scientists work tirelessly to perfect ways to overcome the human immune system in the hopes of one day implanting parts derived from primates or pigs in the bodies of ailing human beings. Such are the futuristic dreams of cutting-edge transplant research. However, whereas the lofty aspirations of mechanical organ design and xenografting each bear promises of saving and extending human lives, associated laboratory and surgical efforts carry complex moral consequences. The moral dimensions of risky experimental science, as expressed by involved practitioners, define the focus of this book.

MORALITY AND THE SCIENTIFIC IMAGINARY

Morality and science are often presumed to define an awkward and even inappropriate pairing because moral thinking hampers scientific pursuits and thus should be the purview of religion and philosophy. Science must remain morally neutral: as philosopher Bernard Rollin (2006) explains, the "logical positivism" of science facilitates the "rejection" or dismissal of "moral discussions as empirically meaningless" (21). This stance is effectively enabled by meticulous adherence to the scientific method, a set of codified practices whose ideological underpinnings insist that science is resolutely objective, unemotional, and, thus, value free (see Rollin 2006, 15–20). Laboratory experiments, for instance, necessitate behaviors that can be replicated by an indeterminate number of personnel; the validity of drug testing is largely dependent on "blind" and even "double blind" procedures; and patterns, measurements, and outcomes are most highly valued when they can be abstracted and quantified. So defined, objectivity eliminates the hazards—or, at the very least, the troublesome noise—of scientists' subjective perceptions, beliefs, and desires.

Throughout *The Transplant Imaginary*, I challenge these assumptions, advocating instead that moral convictions surface regularly in certain scientific domains. Nowhere are such trends more readily apparent than in contexts involving highly experimental and, therefore, conjectural research. As I demonstrate, the realm of experimental human organ replacement offers an especially rich domain in which to explore these ideas. Of special concern to me are efforts to generate alternative sources for allotransplants—that is, organs derived from human donors (both living and dead) that can be transferred to the bodies of patients dying of organ failure. Within barely half a century, allotransplantation has proved to be an enormously successful clinical practice, such that hearts, lungs, livers, pancreases, and kidneys (and over a hundred other reusable human parts) undergo second "lives" when transferred from natal to new (albeit sickly) bodies. Yet the technological inventiveness and prowess that drive this field have proved both blessing and curse, because organs are in increasingly scarce supply as the numbers for patients awaiting transplants grow. Confronted with such social obstacles as widespread public reticence to partitioning bodies for reuse and regulatory apparati that forbid the sale of organs in the majority of countries worldwide, transplant medicine aggressively seeks out other options. This book focuses on two such alternatives to human organ replacement: *biomechanical engineering*, or attempts to design "artificial" or mechanical organs (where heart devices have gained special prominence), and *xenotransplantation*, or efforts to cull organs from "donor" animals (involving simian and, more recently, porcine species).[5]

A key understanding that informs this book is that in contexts framed by highly experimental work—whether in transplant medicine or elsewhere—moral thinking figures prominently in scientific domains, where personal values, training, and experimentation determine scientists' commitments to certain projects over others. Should, for instance, one harness nuclear power for weaponry or for civilian energy needs? Are insects best understood as pests we must eliminate, or should we harvest them as viable protein sources? Are certain research funds, though hefty or lucrative, off-limits because their origins are morally suspect? How should one evaluate the economic, clinical, and social expense of employing various animal species in laboratories? Whose needs should be targeted in one's research—those of infants or the elderly, the wounded or the young and able-bodied, or destitute or paying clients? Is it morally responsible or reprehensible to attempt radically new procedures on or implant experimental devices within terminally ill patients if knowledge garnered from their end-of-life experiences could save others later? And what if these patient-subjects are children? Though muted or undervalued elsewhere, these sorts of questions shape scientists' convictions about the relevance, legitimacy, and social worth of their thoughts, beliefs, and actions when they forge ahead with highly experimental projects.

Moral thinking nevertheless remains obscure in many domains of laboratory science, because attempts to grapple with these sorts of concerns are further troubled by the false premise within associated fields that ethics and morality are synonymous analytical categories.[6] Scientists—be they based in the United States, as I am, or elsewhere—are cognizant of established ethical or "principled" behavior in their respective fields. Scientists I have interviewed regularly frame ethical discussions in reference to codified rules imposed by Institutional Review Boards (IRBs) and federal regulatory agencies (such as the Food and Drug Administration, or FDA): that is, the *bureaucratized*, embedded structures that demarcate (or, as some would argue, restrict) research design and laboratory behaviors.[7] For instance, many contemporary scientists—especially those whose work intersects with clinical medicine—are able to describe with ease the four-principle approach originally conceived by bioethicists Tom Beauchamp and James Childress (1979) emphasizing patient autonomy (and, by association, informed consent), nonmaleficence (inspired by the dictum *primum non nocere* or the imperative of the Hippocratic Oath to do no harm), beneficence (or the obligation to apply one's skills to help others), and justice (such as protecting the rights of others to quality care).

This now widely standardized bioethical framework informs institutionalized rules of professional conduct and research design within government funding agencies, academic settings, and beyond.[8] When bioethics is conflated with morality, it effectively obscures a different sort of logic that may indeed inform scientific interests and decisions, and ultimately determine the trajectory of experimental work beyond the rationale encountered in research proposals and associated evaluations. In an assessment of official reviews of emergent biotechnologies in the United Kingdom, moral philosopher Michael Banner (1999) offers this astute observation: "They demonstrate a tendency to suppose that an ethical analysis of the new technology is exhausted by a prudential consideration of its potential risks and benefits, when this supposition in fact serves to conceal from view many ethical concerns" (207).[9] According to Banner, "the supposedly moral discussion of these issues" exposes conscious efforts by evaluators to deflect contentious relations with science, offering "a satisfactory division of the spoils—that is to say, it makes some concessions to those who would restrain or limit the practice . . . but not such concessions as might seriously hamper either the advance or application of research" (207). I concur with his somewhat cynical assessment: contentious encounters with social activists and others may indeed shape scientists' pursuits in profound ways (Sharp 2011c). My key point here, though, is that bioethical standards (which do promote risk/benefit analyses) not only "conceal" (and thus deny) but also cloud or hinder our own ability to detect broader moral concerns shared by scientists themselves. This is not to say that researchers veer away from or defy assurances outlined in formalized reports as stipulated by regulatory apparati; rather, the domains circumscribed by standardized *bioethical* codes of conduct at times overlap with, yet at still other moments prove surprisingly distinct from, *moral* predicaments that confront scientists in quotidian contexts. My purpose within this book is to uncover the prominence of moral thinking by exploring how involved scientists identify, struggle with, and respond to such predicaments in the day-to-day context of highly experimental laboratory pursuits.

A key concern of *The Transplant Imaginary* is what I reference as *moral thinking in science*, a process that falls beyond codified behaviors circumscribed by the field of formal bioethics. More specifically, my ethnographic work as a medical anthropologist investigates in quotidian contexts why, when, and how scientists imagine and think through the short- and long-term consequences of cutting-edge transplant research directed at nonhuman sources of organ replacement, with the understanding that such "imaginings" might be glossed elsewhere in science as irrelevant because they are too "subjective," "personal," "situational," "emotional," or "private." Because of the weight and greater legitimacy assigned to objective frames of reference, moral thinking is all too often discredited as anecdotal, possibly political, potentially unprofessional, and inevitably unscientific. Yet, as I will argue throughout this study, moral thinking may figure prominently in science, and it can shape in profound ways the trajectories research efforts assume. Furthermore, moral thinking is especially pronounced when scientific work is understood by its practitioners as *highly experimental*, precisely because involved scientists so often imagine their efforts in such contexts as daring ventures into *terra incognita*, an imaginative stance that inspires scientists to contemplate the social and temporal ramifications of what they most desire.

The Transplant Imaginary further postulates that highly experimental research in human organ replacement offers especially fertile ground for such an investigation, one intended to be of comparative value (that is, applicable, at the very least, to other non-transplant-related realms). Organ transplantation presents an ideal context for studying scientific morality precisely because it has long stood as a gold standard in clinical work, ceaselessly blending technical sophistication with medical innovation. Economic, social, and clinical stakes are extraordinarily high within this domain, legitimating especially bold undertakings. In the United States especially, organ replacement is regarded by many as requiring among the most complex and prestigious surgical skills; a hospital's stature may depend on the number of transplant surgeries its staff perform annually; and pronounced shortages in life-saving organs underscore the critical state of transplant medicine. Laboratory-based researchers are acutely aware of these and related factors that then fuel their own daring efforts, such as extending the ex-corporeal life of donated organs so they can survive several hours of transport, enhancing surgical techniques that improve graft survival, perfecting immunosuppressive drug regimens that sustain patients throughout the post-surgical phase of their lives, and generating creative ways to increase organ supply, involving, for instance, trisecting livers, salvaging compromised organs for transplant, or devising new methods of brain-dead donor management. All of these actions are shaped by a pronounced sense of urgency, driven by the paired moral imperatives to alleviate organ scarcity and diminish human suffering.

I have written extensively (Sharp 2006b) on how these moral imperatives—and associated anxieties and desires—shape the trajectory of contemporary organ transfer[10] in the United States. Building on this earlier work, *The Transplant Imaginary* addresses related albeit qualitatively different scientific activities, namely efforts to generate alternatives to organs of human origin such that transplant surgeons might one day bypass altogether the capricious supply of those derived from altruistic strangers, kin, friends, coworkers, and acquaintances who donate parts of themselves to patients dying of organ failure. In this light, xenotransplantation and biomechanical engineering, as radical experimental trajectories, are best understood as forms of *anticipatory science* that bear enormous hope and promise for transplant medicine in the *longue durée* (see Guyer 2007).

Both trajectories lay claim to established histories of experimental work that foreground the importance of transplantation as the hallmark of twentieth (and now twenty-first) century medical expertise. Xenotransplantation began in earnest during the early years of the twentieth century, and bioengineering emerged slightly later, during the interwar years. Although these fields define two distinct—and, now, competing—realms of experimental science, they have developed in tandem, together supplying knowledge leading to significant advancements in allotransplantation, genetics, immunology, animal research, anatomy, and embodied forms of structural design. Interestingly, their respective histories also converge in their shared claims to the inspirational and foundational work of Alexis Carrel. Although Carrel is best known for advancing vascular surgery (for which he was awarded a Nobel Prize), by 1910 he had experimented extensively with xenografting with a range of animal species, and by 1935, in partnership with aviator Charles Lindbergh, he created an early perfusion pump, a device now recognized as a precursor to the heart-lung bypass machine (D. Friedman 2007). As such, xenotransplantation (henceforth *xeno*) and biomechanical engineering (henceforth *bioengineering*) together enable one to track across a full century the moral undertone of professional narratives of the origins, persistence, advancements, and promises of innovative transplant pursuits.

GROUNDINGS

The Transplant Imaginary is informed by several premises. First, it draws inspiration from arguments posited over a decade ago by Mary-Jo DelVecchio Good (2001, see also 2007), who, while studying innovative albeit troubled therapies in oncology, identified the "biotechnical embrace" and the "medical imaginary" as significant "interpretative concepts" (2001, 395–96) and, I would add, interrelated processes.[11] DelVecchio Good raised probing questions about the "imaginary" that are relevant to my own research, asking "how do local and international political economies of medical research and biotechnology shape medicine's scientific imaginary, its cultural, moral and ethical worlds, and the structure of inequalities of use, access and distribution of medicine's cultural and material 'goods'? . . . What form does the 'political economy of hope' take? How do the culture of medicine and the production of bioscience and biotechnology 'live' in respective societies?" (396). For her, "the concept of 'embrace' conjure[s] . . . affective responses," and she demonstrates that clinicians and patients alike "are energized by enthusiasm albeit tempered with irony" in response to "nascent technologies" and the promises and, more important, "hope" they bear for biomedicine's progress (DelVecchio Good 2001, 399; see also Mattingly 2010). In fact, she regards "innovative organ transplantation procedures" as exemplary (DelVecchio Good 2001, 399). I, too, am intrigued by the imaginative processes that inform laboratory research, my project driven by the understanding that the more experimental the pursuit, the more open-ended the imaginative scientific processes might be. Following DelVecchio Good's lead, I assert that the "scientific imaginary" simultaneously shoulders themes of longing, hope, promise, and desire in contexts where the endpoint (or endpoints) remain(s) unknown.

The second premise of this book is that high levels of unpredictability are what stimulate moral thinking in experimental science. Whereas formalized discussions may remain muted or even be actively discouraged in particular contexts (such as press conferences, interviews with reporters, Congressional hearings, regulatory assessments, or IRB reports), my active ethnographic engagement with experimental transplant scientists reveals that moral thinking abounds in a range of other settings. Individual scientists are apt to be more candid in response to moral questions when speaking privately or when consulted in their own laboratories where they claim expertise and control. Moral thinking flourishes, too, in other domains when scientists are among like-minded colleagues. For instance, xeno and bioengineering conferences regularly host plenary sessions and keynote speakers as a means to stimulate lively discussions on a range of broadly defined ethical concerns and social dangers, including zoonotic infections, device malfunction, patients' experiences with social stigma, and the experimental use of human and animal subjects. Within these contexts, participants voice personal and highly subjective points of view. As such, these events also facilitate boundary work that ultimately delimits moral practices and thought.

Third, this project assumes (or, perhaps better phrased, presumes) that quotidian and, thus, mundane scientific practices can reveal much more about the values that drive "science in action" (Latour 1987) than do the codified structures and regulatory apparati of bioethics. That is, whereas formalized bioethical principles help scientists think about what they should or must not do, a focus on moral thinking helps uncover the more imaginative aspects of scientific desires as they unfold in everyday life. Thus, this study recognizes the importance of bioethics in science and, more specifically, in clinical practice, but the much broader (and, I maintain, *more imaginative*) domain of morality offers intriguingly elaborate, sophisticated, deeply nuanced, and alternative readings of how scientists think through and justify what they do in the laboratory and beyond. As I will demonstrate, attention to quotidian contexts exposes subjectivity's vitality in shaping the values—and virtues—of highly experimental pursuits.

When taken together, these premises require radically different social and temporal stances than those that typify ethics statements, progress reports, and linear professional histories. Whereas bioethical frameworks ground research design in assurances made in the past and present about what one promises to do—and not do—in the future (as exemplified by IRB requirements), moral thinking allows scientists greater freedom to think creatively in a mode akin to what Jane Guyer (2007) has identified as the "promissory" imagining of idealized outcomes focused on the distant future (see also Sharp 2011c). For instance, the scientists with whom I work often speak in terms of "what if": What if blood typing no longer mattered and organs and tissues could be shared by any and all bodies? What if we could grow organs from scratch that were tailored to the personal needs and size of individual patients? What if we could render human and chimpanzee tissue compatible and, thus, easily interchangeable? What if we could breed *en masse* hybrid swine to harbor human genetic material so that their organs and tissues would "fool" our immune systems into perceiving them as "self" and not "foreign"? What if a mechanical heart could be as light, efficient, and strong as a patient's fleshy, natal one? What if this heart's power source were fully internalized and required no recharging? What if these innovative procedures and inventions meant we could eliminate altogether the need for donated human parts? In each of these imagined scenarios, scientific creativity is understood not merely as a set of discrete laboratory-based events (when, for example, particular discoveries are "made") but rather as elaborate social and temporal *processes* with multiple destinies and, thus, unfixed futures.

ETHNOGRAPHIC IMAGININGS

Such concerns circumscribe contexts ideally suited to ethnographic inquiry. Anthropology, after all, has long claimed expertise in investigating moral systems, or what Gregory Bateson (1958) referenced long ago as cultural *ethos*. In turn, an especially vigilant focus on quotidian and, therefore, the often mundane aspects of social life defines the very foundation of ethnographic investigations, particularly where the technique of participant-observation is employed. As Bronislaw Malinowski (1922), a founding architect of the field, originally asserted, among "*the imponderabilia of actual life* . . . belong such things as the routine of a man's working day . . . the tone of conversational and social life . . . passing sympathies . . . [and] the subtle yet unmistakable manner in which personal vanities and ambitions are reflected in the behaviour of the individual and in the emotional reactions of those who surround him" (18–19). As readers familiar with this oft-quoted passage already know, Malinowski drew from experiences on Kiriwina in the western Pacific, yet his guidance proves instructive within contemporary scientific contexts, too. After all, he insisted both on scientific rigor and on imaginative data-gathering techniques involving close attention to quotidian actions, beliefs, desires, and emotions. The power of the "ethnographic imagination," as Paul Willis (2000, 6) has argued more recently, lies in its ability to engender awareness of the "possibilities" inherent in the connections between art and everyday life. We may similarly approach scientific experimentation as a creative enterprise or "art," where the "what if" quality of scientists' musings renders visible otherwise indiscernible moral possibilities. For the sake of my own project, the "artists" at work are laboratory-based scientists set on creating innovative procedures and devices that may one day profoundly alter others' everyday existences. When framed as such, experimental science is easily redefined as their craft or domain of artistry.

As noted above, my project emerged from a larger and older body of research that analyzed the social worth of bodies and the theme of self-transformation in the context of human organ transfer in the United States (Sharp 2006b, 2007). This previous research was most intensely concentrated on the transformative properties of cadaveric organ transfer, a simultaneously clinical and social process that generates deeply personal "affective responses" (again, see DelVecchio Good 2001) among transplant recipients and the surviving kin of deceased organ donors. Members of each group must grapple with efforts to distinguish self from other where extraordinary biomedical interventions necessitate the permanent breaching of multiple bodies' boundaries. Involved professionals—be they surgeons, transplant nurses or social workers, or organ procurement specialists—invest significant effort in denying the strange, uncanny, and troubling aspects of organ transfer, a stance facilitated by elaborate forms of rhetorical policing, word play, and metaphorical representations that both objectify fleshy parts and obscure their troubled human origins (Richardson 1996; Sharp 2001; Youngner 1990). In contrast, involved lay parties—most notably transplant recipients and the surviving kin of deceased donors—are alert to the moral consequences of organ transfer, raising questions about the unknown suffering endured by organ donors during the accidents, conditions, and illnesses responsible for their deaths; the economic consequences of post-transplant survival; the murkiness of brain death criteria; and the postmortem histories of deceased persons whose parts have been dispersed to others who reside in one's county, state, or nation.

Early on, I became acutely aware of a longing expressed by members of all parties—both lay and professional—for alternative sources of transplantable parts. This longing sprang from widespread anxieties over the chronic scarcity of human organs. Yet I argue, too, that anxieties over the cadaveric origins of organs (or what Stuart Youngner [1990] has labeled transplant's "dark side") play an equal part in this quest for alternatives. Transplant conferences and other related events nearly always host at least one panel, keynote address, plenary session, or luncheon event designed to address alternative solutions, and xenografts and artificial devices dominate these discussions. Themes of wonder and hope pervade these events, and what might be perceived in other contexts as dry and rather dull technical presentations here signal a strong—and alternative—scientific longing for alleviating human suffering.

I must stress from the very start, however, that this is not a study of patients' experiences. These are still highly experimental domains, and thus my work focuses nearly exclusively on the lives of the scientists intimately involved in these two trajectories of transplant-related research. Within xeno science, there are (to my knowledge) no humans alive whose bodies incorporate whole organs derived from animals, the most recently reported surgeries having been conducted in the 1990s and, further, save for two puzzling anomalies (see chapter 2), experimental patients never survive more than a few hours or, at best, weeks. Bioengineering has proved more successful, especially in the past few years. In fact, over the course of this project I have watched ventricular assist devices (VADs) move from being experimental apparatuses involved in a few small trials scattered across the globe to a technology that might soon become a routinized practice in cardiac wards, especially as a "bridge to transplant" intended to "buy time" (see Copeman 2005) for patients awaiting allografts. Some surgeons now argue that these should be employed as "destination therapy," or permanently implanted, too. Total artificial hearts (TAHs) have suffered from multiple failures, although some models are likewise proving to be extraordinarily promising where, in some cases, patients are being discharged from hospitals and going home with portable drivers in tow in wheelie backpacks. More important, though, clinicians are fiercely protective of their patients' privacy and the confidentiality of research, rendering it exceptionally difficult to gain access to "implantees." Out of respect for these conditions, in addition to FDA and in-house IRB regulations and the like, my own research has excluded patients from the start as a primary social category of analysis.

I do, nevertheless, encounter with startling frequency people who have porcine (and, to a lesser extent, bovine) heart valves, as well as others of a wide range of ages whose bodies bear implanted defibulators. They offer complex stories and insights on the significance of these embodied technologies and the ways that each can radically alter one's sense of self (and, especially with defibulators, the frailty of life, should their heart and device fail simultaneously). I likewise encounter cardiac and thoracic surgeons who implant heart valves, pacemakers, defibulators, and, increasingly, VADs in patients, and their thoughtful critiques on the importance of patient- (versus device-) centered care have taught me much about the complexities that characterize their own lives as caregivers in this era of postmillennial medicine.

That said, parts of animal and mechanical origins are widely perceived by involved experimental scientists as morally neutral: for example, pigs, as farm animals, are already consumed for their meat, and mechanical parts are inert and thus "value free." These sorts of qualities render them superior to parts acquired from human bodies through elaborate systems of informed consent. As a result, xenografting and the bioengineering of artificial organs quickly emerge as processes that are *morally superior* to allotransplantation. Because both xenografts and artificial devices potentially could be mass produced yet also tailor-made, both alternatives could well circumvent chronic problems that plague healthcare access in the United States by crossing barriers of age and size, gender, race and social class, and religious orientation. That is, devices could conceivably be individually engineered to fit any body; domesticated swine could be bred cheaply to provide an unending supply of parts even for the uninsured; and transplant professionals would no longer need to struggle to overcome the moral scruples of surviving kin disturbed by the corporeal disfigurement that cadaveric organ donation entails. Within these imaginative domains, both experimental immunologists and bioengineers emerge as heroic figures who define the vanguard of transplant medicine's future. As such, it is hardly any wonder that their efforts are tracked by venture capitalists (Maeder and Ross 2002) and achieve such honors as *Time*'s "Invention of the Year" award (Hamilton 2001). In these celebratory contexts, the moral traction of the transplant imaginary can be extraordinarily difficult to ignore.

THE EXPERIMENTAL ETHOS AND THE SCIENTIFIC IMAGINATION

Efforts to explore moral frameworks are often plagued by a troublesome paradox of which ethnographers are all too familiar: on the one hand, we seek to identify patterns of thought and behavior; on the other, such an investigation inevitably invites subjective—and, thus, highly individualized—responses. Throughout this project, I have struggled to determine how best to assert both at once. That is, how do scientists based in a range of labs and other settings display comprehensive moral frameworks reflective of their professions and passions? How is one to reconcile the manifestation of a wide array of opinions (and depths of moral sophistication) in work environments where such discussions may not be part of everyday practice, such that they surface only occasionally or haphazardly (see Helmreich 2009; Latour 1999a)? In response to my questions, scientists expressed such sentiments as "engineers prefer to leave the ethical debates to the clinicians" or that science has "no room" for morality. At other moments I have endured tirades against FDA constraints, or listened patiently to seemingly spontaneous yet very detailed philosophical discussions, where key ideas are mapped out so meticulously as to approximate canned sound bites or a well-crafted PowerPoint presentation. What the interviewed scientists share in common, though, is a keen awareness of the complexities associated with the value of human life, the imperative to overcome presumably insurmountable obstacles, the multifaceted nature of suffering, and the emotional impact endured when faced with dying patients (especially when these patients are children). These factors generate widespread moral awareness, which profoundly shapes their professional careers over months, years, and decades of experimental engagement in their laboratories—and beyond.

As Bruno Latour has so convincingly demonstrated, laboratories are not social isolates. His invaluable work underscores that one must heed "the irrelevance of too sharp a distinction between the 'inside' and the 'outside'" of a laboratory's boundaries[12] (1999b, 258). For helpful roadmaps that span the ins and outs of laboratory science, I draw simultaneously on Stefan Helmreich's (2009) work with oceanographers intent on uncovering the mysterious nature of alternative life forms of the deep sea, and that of political philosopher Annemarie Mol (2002), who demonstrates in remarkable ways the multiple routes, moral systems, and bodies that surface and are imagined within a hospital in specific reference to atherosclerosis. These authors' handling of seemingly mundane categories has inspired me to ask similar questions about experimental transplant science: how do scientists frame their understandings of organ replacement, intended patients' bodies, and the technologies their work entails? What are the moral consequences of their professional values and desires? How are such sentiments enacted in the laboratory, professional conferences, and clinical settings? What might be the unintentional consequences of such imaginings? What happens when they encounter patients face-to-face? I hope that the range of positions described within this work will not be viewed as a cacophony of perspectives but will—at the very least—inspire involved scientists and other curious readers to think more broadly and deeply about the relevance of multiplicity to moral frameworks.

Given these circumstances, I feel I must forewarn readers before advancing any further: I seek not to identify moments of consensus (though these do arise) among involved scientists. This is, instead, a much messier project, in that it underscores the polyvalent nature of scientists' thoughts on the moral underpinnings of their research goals, activities, and desires. The issues explored throughout this book are framed simultaneously by themes of wonder and struggle. At times, one encounters clear-cut and carefully constructed narratives; at others, scientists' responses reveal an eclectic cobbling together of moral frameworks drawn from a range of disciplines that may be very specific to an individual scientist's career (where supplementary training might well include the history of science, experimental physics, sociology, or animal rights activism). In short, not all scientists think alike. How, then, to track the shared moral meanings (see Helmreich

Introduction

2009, 25) associated with human-engineered body transformations while privileging individual understandings, too?

As Mol (2002) asserts in her work on the multiple ontologies of the body, "All of these, all at once, all intertwined, all in tension. If reality is multiple, it is also political" (7). If we follow Mol's stance and assume for the moment that the "political" glosses inequalities, disparities, and difference, we begin to see that scientists' moral musings are potentially of great (or grave) social value. In this sense, anthropology is extraordinarily effective because it has long shouldered the weight of the seeming disarray of observations, actions, and opinions. The qualitative methodologies that drive ethnographic inquiry are key, simultaneously insisting on careful documentation of even the most mundane details of daily life, on the suspension of one's judgment of others' moral frameworks, and on a high level of tolerance for an open-ended line of questioning. Anthropologists, in short, capture the subtleties of human thought and action that might otherwise escape detection during quantitative pursuits. Finally, anthropology is at its very core a comparative science. I am a firm believer in the dictum that knowledge of social life is enhanced through contrast, a position that has proved fruitful in the context of this project. Comparisons abound throughout this work. They are most evident as I tack back and forth between domains inhabited by xenotransplant experts and bioengineers. Yet other axes are equally important: although my earlier work on organ transfer was based nearly exclusively in the United States (Sharp 2006b), the research that informs *The Transplant Imaginary* led me to four additional Anglophone countries (Canada, the United Kingdom, Australia, and New Zealand), where scientists from both fields viewed one another as members of seamless research cultures yet where nationally instigated regulatory apparati nevertheless informed moral codes of conduct. Still another axis of comparison has involved thinking carefully about individual (or private) versus collective (or profession-based) values, alongside insider or specialist knowledge versus outsider or lay (and, especially, social activist) understandings of the value, necessity, challenges, and dangers of experimentation. Although such musings may seem obvious and even picayune to any anthropologist who reads this, the significance of qualitative, comparative approaches is less obvious among the scientists with whom I have worked, and thus I offer these comments in partial defense of the ethnographic enterprise. Indeed, I am often asked by non-anthropologists *how* I was able to uncover certain findings; I grant credit to a discipline sensitive to other ways of knowing the world as crucial to any success I might claim. The rewards are manifest in the frequency with which scientists articulate their private perceptions of their work, alongside hopes that their efforts might prove socially transformative in the near or distant future.

Inevitably, this project has required moving from the collective to the subjective and back to the collective again. This means, though, that I supply no easy answers or set of recommendations in this book's concluding chapter. Rather, my purpose here is to encourage a fresh sensitivity to the significance of experimental work, generate new ways of thinking more precisely about the moral parameters of futuristic goals within transplant medicine, and alert naïve yet inquisitive readers, alongside seasoned scientific researchers, to the sociomoral complexities of these experimental worlds. My ultimate goal is thus a rather lofty one: How might we shift the frame of reference such that discussions become less about *how* we must pursue these experimental forms of body repair and more about *why* we insist this must be so? Just as Helmreich (2009) interrogates how "sentiment and science about the sea inflect one another" (19) within the field of marine biology, I am intrigued by the sentimental qualities that drive moral thinking among experimental transplant scientists. The answers are complicated, where variation hinges largely on the inevitable subjective nature of the question of what makes for a moral science.

Throughout this work, I grant special weight to themes of wonder and conviction that at times encourage, legitimate, and drive, and, at others, forestall scientists' struggles to alter a specialized domain of human experience where life and death, survival and failure, and sickness and what Cheryl Mattingly (2010) identifies as the "paradoxes of hope" within "clinical borderlands" all hang in the balance. In certain ways, this is an anthropological study in the extreme, for the discipline is steadfastly tolerant of difference, a theme on which I intend to capitalize. As an ethnographer, I have been trained to seek out patterns of similarity, yet I am also wary of efforts to exclude data (be they categories of people, opinions, or behaviors) that more quantitatively oriented disciplines might disregard or discard as exceptions, "outliers," or statistically irrelevant "noise." My approach is informed in part by a similar tolerance for serendipity within the field known as Science and Technology Studies (STS, henceforth *science studies*). To return to Latour (1999a), boundary work within science (and laboratories) is hardly a neat or linear affair; rather, it involves complex processes marked simultaneously by imaginative conjecture and skilled negotiation. Similarly, I am deeply interested in these negotiative processes that define, in Latour's words, the "black box" of science (1999a). This is especially pertinent, I argue, given that the endpoint(s) for experimental transplant research have yet to be reached and are thus, at best, highly speculative. Entering the field at this point—be it as an ethnographer, scientist, clinician, or, for that matter, patient—is simultaneously exciting, disorienting, frightening, perplexing, and wondrous. A desire that drives my own work, then, is to try to convey this sense of excitement and wonder in my efforts to disentangle the associated complex of moral quandaries so central to experimental, conjectural science.

Finally, ethnography enables one to uncover moral systems as part and parcel of larger social processes. Throughout *The Transplant Imaginary*, I seek to trace how scientists talk informally about their work in quotidian contexts. Moral values are evident not merely in their words but also in their actions, the material culture they produce, and the visual representations of their work. Whereas I most certainly owe a heavy debt to science studies, I am far less interested in discrete "enactments" involving "actors" and "actants"[13] than I am in deciphering the deeper meanings expressed by scientists as they think through and try to articulate what it is they strive to do in their transplant-inspired work. Serious moral consequences are at stake here, concerning the genetic hybridization of species, the technological enhancement of the human form, and the physical and psychological harm endured by experimental animal and human subjects, as well as more general questions regarding the prioritization of healthcare needs across diverse populations. As such, this is no mere exercise in ethnographically inspired philosophy.[14] Rather, it is a concerted attempt to uncover what scientists themselves think they are doing as a means, in turn, to inspire them to reflect more broadly and deeply on the complexity of what is at stake as they toil away in the seclusion of their laboratories.

THE HISTORY OF A PROJECT

This project emerged slowly out of a wider interest and involvement in organ transfer in the United States that spanned 1991–2004. Discussions of transplant's future were so common during professional gatherings that, when the topic was excluded from conference programs and the like, I would find myself wondering if the organizers lacked vision. At times, presenters made wild claims about transplantation's potential; more often, though, discussions were unquestionably driven by deep-set anxieties over the nation's seemingly growing scarcity of organs. In such contexts, organs were even described as a scarce national resource, where the trope of scarcity bore an eerie resemblance to narratives in radically different contexts about oil reserves, water rights, and land development in other professional quarters of the country. Within a decade, this discourse of organ scarcity had spread abroad: during international transplant conferences, presenters from such diverse origins as Mexico, Canada, England, Denmark, Australia, New Zealand, Japan, China, Singapore, Turkey, India, and Brazil would rely on turns of phrase that had undoubtedly originated with the American transplant industry. In fact, it was not unusual for professionals from other countries or agencies (including the World Health Organization, in one instance) to cite statistics from the United Network for Organ Sharing (UNOS)—which is based in Richmond, Virginia, is funded in large part by Congress, and oversees the fair distribution of organs exclusively within the United States—as if its efforts represented global trends. These same speakers regularly embraced xeno, bioengineering, and, to a lesser extent, tissue engineering as the future's viable, lifesaving alternatives.

By 2003, I had embarked on exploratory research focused on the potentialities of these futuristic visions. Gradually, this project grew into a study focused on interrelated activities of xeno specialists and bioengineers based in five Anglophone countries: the United States, Canada, the United Kingdom, Australia, and New Zealand. Although scattered across the globe, specialists from these countries express often remarkably similar—and thus generalizable—moral tendencies, where shared ideas and associated turns of phrase spring in part from similar (and postwar) bioethical frameworks that define the mainstay of scientific regulatory apparati. Whereas longstanding relationships with colleagues from other nations (most notably continental

Europe, China, Taiwan, Japan, and Singapore) are equally significant within both fields, overlapping moral convictions regarding the treatment of human and animal subjects led me to focus exclusively on Anglophone contexts. Significant linguistic and cultural barriers (for me as well as for involved scientists of a range of nationalities) play a partial role in maintaining such a divide. I should note, however, that these five countries are widely regarded within each profession as leading global sites of innovation.

When I initiated this project, the new trajectory offered relief, too, from research fatigue within a medical realm where one encounters death at nearly every turn. In retrospect, I realize that I was not unlike the very scientists whom I sought to investigate, in that I, too, would spend time in laboratories, naïvely imagining I would be insulated from the suffering endured by patients and their family members. Yet suffering emerged once again as an essential focus for analysis, defining a paradoxical absent presence (Jensen 2010) over the course of the following eight years of involvement. Tragic stories of loss and endless mourning characterized the world of cadaveric donation (where the stories told by surviving donor kin destabilized the upbeat messages of hope and rebirth promoted by transplant professionals). In stark contrast, I soon found that immunologists and bioengineers were often so focused on the microscopic, inert, or nonhuman aspects of their work as to bracket out the suffering of patients (and, for that matter, of the animal subjects housed in their laboratories).[15] I learned that their research is instead about *eliminating* suffering in the distant future by overcoming myriad obstacles and deficiencies that characterize the present reliance on donated allografts. Thus, it is not that these scientists are unaware of suffering, or that suffering is absent from their professional discourse; rather, suffering occupies a very different moral register, one framed by the drive to eliminate organ scarcity altogether.

The settings and contexts that define the parameters of this research are diverse. They include personal visits to individual researchers' laboratories, on-site engagements at corporate headquarters, individual interviews with scientists ranging from seniors in the field to burgeoning graduate and undergraduate students, and attendance at a wide array of conferences in the United States, Canada, England, Australia, and New Zealand. Professional conferences have proved to be especially rich sites for this particular project, because it is at these moments that otherwise fairly isolated laboratory researchers gather to compare notes, present their data, and compete with one another, too, over the intricacies of knowledge relevant to device design, the human/animal immunological interface, the anatomical barriers of the fleshy body, and the ethics of research strategies and goals. Over the course of nearly eight years, I attended six annual conferences of bioengineers sponsored by the American Society for Artificial Internal Organs (ASAIO), which claims to be the oldest transplant association in existence; two separate meetings of Medicine Meets Virtual Reality, an eclectic group of clinical, engineering, artificial intelligence, animation, and haptics experts; five other international transplant conferences (more often frequented by xeno experts and not bioengineers); and a sixth that was dedicated exclusively to xenotransplantation. These venues offered an invaluable approach for tracking the progress of (and shifts in) ongoing research over time while also granting easy access to key players in the fields relevant to my research. Leaders within both disciplines are eager to foster the progress of a younger and fresh generation of scientists, and thus, again, it was most often at these professional gatherings that I encountered students at all levels from a range of laboratories, universities, and countries, the majority of whom think carefully about morality and virtuousness in science (quite often in more sophisticated ways than their senior mentors).[16]

Within this book, I consider four moral domains: the ways in which the human body is reconfigured and imagined in highly experimental contexts; the promises, challenges, and dangers of embodied hybridity and interspeciality; the presumed perfection associated with artificial, mechanical design; and the temporal framing of scientific desire. Each of these themes defines the focus of a discrete chapter. Thus, chapter 1, "The Reconfigured Body of the Transplant Imaginary," interrogates the premise that experimental work necessitates tampering with the body's integrity, where involved subjects include both animals and humans. The use of bodies is essential to testing experimental ideas; because it also induces harm, involved scientists must think with care about the moral parameters of their work. I am interested in how standardized bioethical frameworks inflect sometimes individualized sentiments and convictions. More important, though, are scientists' quotidian behaviors and sentiments: these expose all too frequently overlooked—yet richly textured—moralities. Within such contexts, one encounters the logic of experimental work regarding efforts to fabricate (and legitimate) human bodies composed in part of artificial and animal parts.

In chapter 2, "Hybrid Bodies and Animal Science: The Promises of Interspecies Proximity," I explore the first of two ethnographic domains central to this project. Although efforts within xeno science correspond with watershed moments in allotransplantation, xeno research has nevertheless been stymied by repeated clinical failures (patients die very soon after implantation) and public resistance (most notably from animal activists). Indeed, one might argue that this pairing of scientific failure with social controversy renders xeno the more highly experimental of the two domains. Such realities shape scientists' moral frameworks in profound ways. Of special import are shifting views on whether simian or porcine species define the most ideal candidates as "donor" species. Categories of experimental animals are imagined differently across species and over time, exposing shifting moral premises regarding the scientific legitimacy of using various creatures in effort to save and extend human lives.

Chapter 3, "Artifical Life: Perfecting the Mechanical Heart," focuses on the second ethnographic domain of bioengineering. Of special concern is how inventors seek to transform the human form, perfecting the flaws of the natal (and, thus, fallible and fleshy) body through biomechanical enhancements, a process often referred to as "tinkering" (Bock and Goode 2007; Mol et al. 2010). This chapter examines what constitutes moral or virtuous behavior in a field where many scientists, if asked directly, assert that ethics is the domain of the clinician and not the engineer. As I will demonstrate, however, engineers' often historicized discourse and behaviors reflect complex moral understandings of what it means to "tinker" with the body and alter its natural form. Those who venture beyond the laboratory and into the clinic also express profound shifts in moral reasoning about what they do, particularly if they encounter patients implanted with the very devices that they themselves have helped design.

Chapter 4, "Temporality and Social Desire in Anticipatory Science," addresses the significance of temporal thinking in experimental domains. Inspired by Jane Guyer (2007), who offers provocative ways to explore temporal discourse, I consider scientists' futuristic ideas as defining an open-ended form of prophecy focused on an ever shifting endpoint. For example, a truism often voiced by xeno researchers is that xeno is "the future of transplantation . . . and always will be" (a statement coined by Sir Roy Calne [2005], a liver surgeon and pioneer within multiple branches of transplant research). Bioengineers, in contrast, often underscore that their work is never truly completed, because every prototype has design flaws or can always be further refined or perfected. In their various efforts, xeno scientists and bioengineers must each rely on the steady flow of investment capital, inevitably transforming animals, heart devices, and human patients, too, into potentially lucrative sources of biocapital. The fickleness of venture capital has an especially profound effect on the trajectory of research for each of these domains—shaping, in turn, a calculus of life and death in the clinic.

In the book's concluding chapter, "The Moral Parameters of Virtuous Science," I circle back to these earlier discussions, revisiting questions of longing as a means to address the inseparable values of desire, hope, and compassion in two experimental domains whose experts are intent on radically transforming the human body and life itself.

CHAPTER ONE

The Reconfigured Body of the Transplant Imaginary

The transplant imaginary is very much a moral domain. Surgeons, patients, health activists, and many in the general populace understand human organ transfer as beleaguered by intense shortages, where the gap between supply and demand increases each year. Transplant specialists are driven nevertheless by the desire to alleviate human suffering by replacing patients' diseased organs with those derived from other bodies, pushing ever higher the number of patients on waiting lists for replacement parts. These surgeries have become so commonplace in some hospitals as to generate a discourse of patients' rights among those who suffer from acute or chronic—and often inevitably terminal—forms of organ failure. The field itself is readily and widely imagined as plagued by unwarranted suffering, where concerns may focus nearly exclusively on the needs of dying patients yet not, for instance, on broader health disparities that shape the calculus of heart or lung disease, liver failure, or diabetes, on the circumstances of donors' sudden or even violent deaths, or on the often insurmountable, lifetime costs accompanying the promise of a "second life" won through the transplantation of a new organ. When framed this way, organ transfer is rife with "if only" statements: if only there were more willing donors; if only presumed consent legislation could prevail; if only viable, alternative sources existed for scarce human body parts.

These sorts of "if only" or "what if" statements lay bare professionals' anxieties that then drive the transplant imaginary. As Thomas O. Beidelman (1993) has detailed, the "moral imagination" as a social process materializes during moments marked by confusion and cultural dissonance. A hallmark of the moral imagination is its open-endedness, where resolution may prove impossible or even seem irrelevant. Beidelman examines the particulars of this process within Kaguru society in East Africa, demonstrating how discordant events, eccentric behaviors, and provocative mythological creatures stimulate moral questioning and debate. Although some readers here might regard Kaguru sentiments irrelevant to their own lives, one need only consider recent works by Julie Livingston (2005, 2012) on debility and oncology in southern Africa, or Mary-Jo DelVecchio Good's (2001) research within an oncology ward in the United States, to grasp the elegance of Beidelman's notion of the imaginary and how beautifully it translates to both clinical and laboratory contexts. Indeed, one encounters significant overlap in these seemingly disparate domains. Be it limited services for the homebound, the unknown outcomes of new treatments for cancer patients, or the shortage of transplantable parts for those dying of organ failure, unpredictability, uncertainty, and the unknown are quotidian aspects of life. These sorts of circumstances inspire moral reasoning and the politics of hope.

Throughout *The Transplant Imaginary*, I strive to "surface" (Taylor 2005)—so as to probe and analyze—the "affective dimensions" (DelVecchio Good 2001) of two morally provocative "clinical borderlands" (Mattingly 2010). The richness of the transplant imaginary is facilitated by its highly experimental nature, where scientists at work on either xenografting or artificial organ design must embrace as givens that research outcomes are open-ended, that future successes are difficult to predict, and that the experimental process presents extraordinary challenges at nearly every turn. Some might go so far as to say that involved researchers are at work on the impossible, yet they forge ahead even when confronted with constant failure. Perhaps a device is plagued by coagulation problems; immune system responses to foreign tissue are persistently "hyper-acute"; lab researchers disagree on which design is best; or citizens' groups successfully push through legislation that blocks further research. Scientists in both domains are nevertheless united by the shared conviction that alternative organ replacement is a life and death matter, their imaginations fueled by a persistent longing to eliminate organ scarcity and human suffering. In those instances where "if only" and "what if" questions arise, they imagine alternative futures infused with such moral sentiments as suffering, hope, and experimental desire (see Sharp 2009).

DOMAINS OF SCIENTIFIC DESIRE

Xenografts and bioengineered devices currently dominate the transplant imaginary, and today no gathering of associated specialists is complete without the staging of lively discussions and plenary events that promote the promissory nature of these two highly experimental alternatives. Efforts from within xeno science and bioengineering dominate transplant-related discussions regarding imagined near and distant futures (Guyer 2007); in turn, they have also informed and responded to celebrated advancements in allografting. Both xeno and bioengineering, for instance, have long defined fertile ground for testing various procedures in animal models before attempting them in humans, with surgical efforts extending back a full century. These two fields also boast overlapping professional genealogies: for instance, Alexis Carrel—perhaps best known for his breakthroughs in vascular surgery—was deeply involved in transspecies grafting at the onset of the twentieth century; only a few decades later, he designed an important precursor to the heart-lung bypass machine with aviator Charles Lindbergh (D. Friedman 2007), a partnership I will investigate more thoroughly in chapter 3.

The foundational knowledge that informs the transplant imaginary is inextricably linked to efforts made within these two experimental domains. For instance, all surgeons who are regarded as founding ancestors of organ transplantation engaged at some point during their careers in xenotransplant research as well. Prior to the first successful kidney transfer between identical twins in Boston in 1954, numerous similar surgeries were attempted involving sheep, dogs, and a range of primates. As I will demonstrate in chapter 2, the 1960s define an especially active experimental period, when organs derived from sacrificed chimpanzees were transferred to the bodies of several deathly ill humans. (Needless to say, few of these patients survived for very long following such radical surgeries.) In turn, a wide assortment of artificial (and primarily excorporeal) devices designed by engineers regularly assist clinical efforts to sustain patients awaiting transplants. Whereas a hemodialyzer, ventilator, VAD, and even surgically employed bypass machine are all understood by involved surgeons as effective "bridges" to transplant and thus as temporary forms of life support, bioengineers celebrate these same devices as innovative "artificial" kidneys, lungs, and hearts that can augment or even fully replace diseased natal organs. This alternative logic informs engineers' ongoing efforts to refashion, reinvent, and miniaturize a wide range of experimental hardware that could be fully implanted in human bodies as "destination" or permanent therapies. These innovations could render patients ambulatory and free from cumbersome alternatives that currently necessitate being tethered to much larger—and often immobile—machinery as they struggle to stay alive in anticipation of a transplant.

As I seek to demonstrate in this current chapter, moral thinking abounds in transplant research, although it follows different paths among involved xeno experts and bioengineers. A premise that drives my work is that moral thinking, though frequently downplayed or silenced, is intrinsic to scientific decision making, and this is especially true in research domains that are highly experimental. As Thomas Kuhn (1962) so adeptly argued half a century ago, the formulation and, in turn, acceptance of scientific ideas as "truths" together emerge through a dialectical process involving sometimes quite prolonged periods of contestation, struggle, and crisis that might later generate paradigmatic shifts. If, in following Kuhn, one embraces the notion that dynamism rather than stasis characterizes scientific inquiry, then those endeavors understood as highly experimental might well be viewed as science in hyperdrive. This is not because the associated laboratory work itself is fast-paced (in fact, to an outsider its progress may seem sluggish at best). Yet the shifting quality of ideas, theories, and relevant outcomes are by very definition in a state of flux during highly experimental pursuits, and this is especially true when work is suffused with personal doubt, potentially insurmountable technical obstacles, a shortage of investment capital, and broader social concerns or, even, disapproval. In these contexts, ideas constantly undergo rigorous redesign, retesting, and reanalysis, only to loop back and start again in response to evolving challenges, flaws, and failures. In other words, experimental science is at its heart a tentative enterprise. I maintain that these sorts of conditions engender an especially ripe environment for moral thinking precisely because theories and outcomes—set alongside their intrinsic social value—have yet to gel.

If transplant medicine itself is driven by "if only" desires, xeno and bio-engineering research are framed by questions of "what if": What if we could circumvent the need for human organs? What if the immune system could read animal flesh as human? What if a fully implantable mechanical device could function as well as or exceed the abilities of a natal organ? The broadest response would be that potentially all patients could then be guaranteed a second lease on life. These imaginings focus simultaneously on contemporary suffering and on the promises of science in the *longue durée*. In turn, they transform experimental work into a moral enterprise precisely because outcomes are subject on some level to conjecture, and thus they remain indeterminate and obscure. Barbara Koenig, writing of the "technological imperative" in biomedicine (1988), demonstrates how in American settings bioethical thinking is muted or neglected and then rendered obsolete once technological innovations become routinized clinical practices. In contrast, I argue that moral thinking abounds in domains marked by apprehension, doubt, and uncertainty, and perhaps nowhere is this more prevalent than during highly experimental phases of scientific research.

A key question, of course, is what counts as morality or, more precisely, moral thinking in science? (For the moment I conflate the terms "morality" and "ethics," only to draw distinctions between these later.) My investigation of scientific morality was originally inspired in large part by Paul Brodwin's earlier work (2000) on the ethical parameters of biotechnologies.[1] Although Brodwin and his coauthors devote much of their attention to encounters with biotechnologies within primarily noncosmopolitan settings, Brodwin's approach is equally relevant to the very scientists responsible for designing such technologies. As he demonstrates, anxieties uncover, mark, accompany, and generate ethical thinking regarding biotechnical interventions, and his method of framing has taught me as an ethnographer to pay close attention to those moments when subjects' anxieties surface.

As I learned during earlier work on human organ transfer, sometimes the richest data emerge at moments of fracture, contestation, paradox, doubt, and debate. I offer this important caveat, however: I am not proposing that one root out disagreements in search of compelling data. Instead, it is the unpredictable and serendipitous nature of such moments that renders them so interesting, especially in regard to sentiments that run contrary to orthodox ideas—or what Pierre Bourdieu (1994) identifies as *doxa*. This is where moral thinking abounds. As moral thinking "surfaces" (Taylor 2005), it reveals richly textured yet otherwise obscured facets of a scientific imagining of the sociomoral parameters of transplant research, the ethical use of human and animal subjects, the boundaries of the "natural" body, and the promissory qualities assigned to futuristic medical pursuits.

If paradox, contestation, and debate are intrinsic to the transplant imaginary, how then might moral thinking be identified and categorized? Among the greater hurdles to such an investigation is that contradictory moral frameworks can, and often do, coexist in experimental science, not only because they predate and inform paradigmatic shifts but also because xeno and bioengineering each encompasses a wide array of disciplines (including virology, immunology, veterinary medicine, surgery, structural engineering, fluid dynamics, and bioartificial design). Moral thinking across these two domains is therefore extraordinarily complex precisely because the ground beneath is varied and, further, is constantly shifting.

Like Bruno Latour, I am deeply intrigued by the "circulating reference[s]" (1999a) that, in this instance, flag moral thinking. As we shall see, these include the values assigned to body integrity, human and animal subjects, technologies of human design, and even time itself. Just as a dedicated astrophysicist might also be a devout Catholic, so too might a xeno researcher assert certain principles of animal sentience and pain sensation while still employing a range of intelligent creatures in his or her research; elsewhere this same scientist might oppose colleagues' use of certain mammalian species over others in the name of scientific rigor. Similarly, a bioengineer might celebrate the inventiveness of a pulseless artificial heart whereas others regard this same innovation as inherently unnatural, physiologically dangerous, and unfit for human use. I offer these examples as evidence not of confusion or hypocrisy within these two fields but, rather, of the variegated nature of corresponding moral values.

As my research reveals, individual experimental scientists may well move freely and comfortably across different moral registers. If asked point blank to discuss the significance of morality in science, common responses include silence or puzzlement; yet elaborately complex answers emerge when scientists describe the sociomedical value of their research, their

efforts to justify their work to nonspecialists, or why they persevere knowing that their work may not reach fruition in their own lifetimes. Those
whom I have interviewed regularly provide thoughtful—and thought-provoking—answers to how they think about the social value of such work (or,
as activists I have interviewed prefer to phrase it, how they manage to sleep
at night, knowing what they do). Given the wide array of responses, it can be
difficult to follow the anthropological rubric for detecting patterns of
thought and behavior. Yet what most intrigues me about xeno and bioengineering as realms of experimental science is not the either/or of competing
sentiments (that is, what one should or should not do) but, instead, the complex, contradictory ideas that emerge from the spaces that lie in between
these sentiments (see Brodwin 2013). As I will demonstrate later in the two
subsequent chapters, this in-betweeness signals a serious grappling with
moral ideas, spurred on by (though perhaps sometimes sublimated) anxieties about the sociomoral value and consequences of projects intent on
transforming human bodies in unquestionably radical ways.

ETHICAL TURNS

An investigation of "morality" or "moral thinking" in science poses certain
kinds of problems within domains whose practitioners are intent on bracketing out morality. As scientists from a range of disciplines inform me,
"morality" is the purview of religion and philosophy and has no place within
science, a sentiment inevitably exacerbated in the United States, at least, by
highly polarized evolutionist/creationist debates that arise in some quarters.
I nevertheless maintain that scientists regularly frame their work in moral
terms, and that experimental contexts often instill heightened moral alertness. If efforts within experimental transplantation are driven by the desire
to alleviate human suffering, then such work is framed from the very start as
a moral enterprise.

My investigation overlaps with what some identify as the relatively new
"ethical turn" in anthropology (Faubion 2011; Fischer 2001; Heintz 2009;
Howell 1997; Laidlaw 2002; Lambek 2010; Zigon 2008), involving efforts to
move beyond a longstanding interest in moral systems (a foundational concern in anthropology) employed as a means to detect "normative" and, thus,
established systems of thought and behavior.[2] In contrast, those whose

scholarship informs the ethical turn perceive morality not as a static category but as a dynamic social process, and associated authors focus most keenly on moments where moral predicaments arise (see especially Heintz 2009, 1-19; Howell 1997; Zigon 2008). Yet another concern involves probing how moral philosophy itself might enrich the ethnographic enterprise (and, as philosopher Michael Banner's recent work [forthcoming] demonstrates, how anthropological theory and ethnographic methods might inform moral philosophy; see also Mol 2008; Pols 2012). Whether such an approach within anthropology itself is indeed new is debatable: one need only consider the joint effort of May and Abraham Edel (1959) to encounter a much earlier attempt to wed anthropology to philosophy.[3] Nevertheless, central to the ethical turn are questions regarding how individuals make moral decisions and what it means to be a moral person within particular cultural contexts. Certain overarching concerns drive such work, and I summarize these briefly below before I delve into my own project.

First and foremost, human beings are understood as inherently moral creatures who live and cooperate with one another across fields of experience. Anthropologists have long been intrigued by codes of conduct—or those diffuse institutions that fall under such labels as "culture," "law and society," "social structure," and "ethos" and that may simultaneously pervade social, economic, and political spheres. James Laidlaw (2002) and others (see Zigon 2008; Faubion 2011) readily acknowledge the influential pull of Emile Durkheim in fostering this approach, one that has long been a bedrock for much of British, French, and American anthropological analyses of moral systems.[4] According to Laidlaw, Durkheim's writings and influence "reveal the disabling consequences of identifying the social with the moral as he did. Durkheim's 'social' is, effectively, Immanuel Kant's notion of the moral law, with the all-important change that the concept of human freedom, which was of course central for Kant, has been neatly excised from it" (312). As Laidlaw insists, anthropologists are bogged down by the weight of Durkheim's legacy, remaining unimaginative where conflict, dilemmas, transformation, or personal agency are concerned (313; see also Heintz 2009, 2). In response, Laidlaw and others probe ethical behavior and action not in pursuit of established principles and values but as evidence of social processes, where moral behavior emerges from turmoil, confusion, and contradiction, and where, for Laidlaw in particular, agentive acts and associated "freedom" are possible (322; after Foucault 1984). Furthermore, outcomes may not be clear and neat but messy and open-ended. Monica Heintz (inspired by Laidlaw) similarly explains, "moralities are entangled within social action and as such are difficult to pinpoint and analyze" (2009, 3). Evidence of this is most likely to surface when studied ethnographically (Laidlaw 2002, 322; see also Lambek 2010), an extraordinarily important point to which I return below.

Though not readily acknowledged in this recent literature, similar concerns are indeed detectable in early ethnographic projects. Whereas Laidlaw regards Bronislaw Malinowski (1926) as a notable exception—thereby faulting the discipline for its lack of both a "sustained debate" on morality and a "sustained dialogue with moral philosophy" (Laidlaw 2002, 311, 312)—a range of canonical scholarship nevertheless demonstrates anthropological interest not simply in morality but in moral conflict. Margaret Mead (1935) and Ruth Benedict (1934), for instance, both wrote widely about outliers and misfits in Austronesian and Native American contexts, as did Durkheim even earlier ([1897] 1997) in his work on suicide in France. E. E. Evans-Pritchard (1937), in turn, targeted moral dilemmas when he documented efforts among Azande to detect and counteract subversive acts of sorcery, and Gregory Bateson's (1958) framing of *eidos* and *ethos* in his analysis of Iatmul Naven rituals anticipated current efforts by more than half a century. Max Gluckman (1963) and Victor Turner (1967) also generated important scholarship regarding moral responses to conflict, the former addressing the Mau Mau insurgency in colonial Kenya, the latter regarding what to do with a deeply troubled—and troublesome—Ndembu patient in what is now Zambia. In other words, morality tales abound in the anthropological canon, though they may remain undetected because they have not been labeled as such. Whereas one could claim that, in each case, these foundational authors strove to identify clear pathways to social equilibrium or, at the very least, temporary harmony, all also reveal that moral dilemmas have long captivated anthropologists and how morality itself can be a very complex and even unresolvable affair. If this literature tells us anything at all, it is that morality—as social thought, action, and process—defines a domain worthy of more focused anthropological attention.

Those who claim the mantle of the ethical turn frequently argue for the enrichment of anthropology by drawing on an established canon within moral philosophy itself.[5] I am not so interested, however, in promoting a particular philosophical framework as I am with the much broader question of what qualifies as or exemplifies moral thinking and action in two related scientific contexts. As I have discovered, scientists themselves express sometimes wildly different principles steered by highly divergent moral compasses. They are, in short, highly eclectic. Among a host of specialists, I have encountered, for instance, utilitarian, existentialist, libertarian, humanist, Hindu, Jewish, and Catholic arguments for why certain pursuits are moral and others are not, and even individual scientists sometimes provide a dizzying array of ideas that might well exemplify contradictory philosophical frameworks (simultaneously embracing, for instance, universalist principles of the sanctity of the body while insisting on its commodification). Competing political sentiments muddy the waters even more: within a single lab, conference panel, or organization, one meets libertarians, leftist social reformers, and hawkish militarists. As an ethnographer, I recognize that varying sentiments offer evidence not of moral confusion (or ineptitude) but, rather, of the complexities involved in determining how best to practice virtuous science long before successful outcomes are in sight. That is, while working in highly experimental contexts, involved scientists must envision or imagine a host of futures—or what Nikolas Rose (2007) identifies as the inevitability of "multiple histories" (252)—and, in so doing, devise fairly flexible moral principles that assuage their struggles with the unknown.

Yet another source of confusion is the language of the ethical turn. A significant impediment concerns the frequent elision of "morality" with "ethics," a strategy borrowed from moral philosophy itself, where the two terms are often used interchangeably. Anthropologists engaged in the ethical turn have made several attempts to delineate differences between the two, most often employing "morals" to circumscribe normative behavior (that is, what, in any given cultural field, defines what one ought to do), whereas "ethics" designates a more serendipitous process of moral decision making, especially in those instances when actors are faced with contradictions that demand moral consideration. Sadly, though, there is little agreement here, and at times these terms, and their definitions, are *reversed*. In light of this, allow me to clarify what I mean when I speak of morality in science.

The Bioethical Conundrum

Studying questions of morality specifically within transplant-related domains is complicated by the presence of bioethics. Today, bioethics asserts a rather comprehensive presence within science and especially laboratory-based research, proffering a set of universalist principles that guide (and even dictate) what one may or may not do with or to both human and animal subjects. During the course of my interviews with scientists, bioethics surfaced regularly: when I would describe the focus of my research, "moral concerns" were rapidly converted into a set of solid, and highly static, categories most reminiscent of Tom Beauchamp and James Childress's (1979) four-principle approach—known as *principlism*—involving autonomy, nonmaleficence, beneficence, and justice.[6] If we follow Laidlaw's argument that anthropology is hampered by its preoccupation with normative codes of conduct, biomedicine and related domains of scientific research are hopelessly hemmed in by this strident set of four principles. Interestingly, the scientists I encountered generally proved well-versed in this approach,[7] one that then shapes rigorously imposed requirements for grant applications within public and private foundations and universities, alongside now ubiquitous online training and certification programs (especially in the United States). The beauty of this method is its universalism (human subjects are entitled to certain rights and protections across a range of fields) and simplicity (involving a neat set of terms that are easy to remember). Most intriguing is the ever-widening reach of a discipline that is only a few decades old. In addition, I was surprised by the ubiquitous application of the four bioethical principles to science based not only in the United States but also in Canada, the United Kingdom, New Zealand, and Australia. This would not have been the case as recently as fifteen years ago. In other words, bioethics (at least in the guise of the model originally espoused by Beauchamp and Childress) is now pervasive, referencing codified and thus standardized or established categories that dictate moral conduct in the laboratory and beyond.

This is precisely what I am *not* interested in pursuing in the course of this volume; therefore, I myself use "ethics" exclusively to refer to bioethical principles. (I will be careful to specify those instances where I cite authors who use "ethics" and "morality" interchangeably.) Whereas bioethics most certainly clarifies what one must or must not do with human and animal subjects and, further, how one needs to justify one's research in terms of medical and social outcomes, my own line of questioning instead concerns the "what if" quality of the transplant imaginary as focused intently on a prophetic future. My research asks more open-ended questions, such as: What sorts of social transformations do xeno scientists long for in their efforts to generate interspeciality? What values inform decisions to employ a chimp, baboon, or pig as an ideal "source" or "donor" animal? What renders the body more natural or unnatural when whole "natal" organs are excised and replaced by "artificial" parts of human design? What sorts of celebrations, accomplishments, dilemmas, confusion, and suffering inform scientists' values regarding the lives of patients who will someday embody animal organs or mechanized replacement parts? And why pursue xeno science or bioengineering at all when their long-term consequences remain unclear?

This line of questioning is a far cry from the four-pronged bioethical approach of autonomy, nonmaleficence, beneficence, and justice. Although principlism provides a neat analytical framework, I am far more intrigued by the messier circumstances involving sometimes unsolvable dilemmas, or those processes that Beidelman (1993) has described as the workings of the "moral imagination," a domain comprising human efforts to achieve clarity in the face of disruption, disorder, paradox, or bewilderment (see also Zigon 2008). Whereas Beidelman tracks how moral thinking responds to adversity and even to those contexts where resolution may be impossible (see Livingston 2005), his framework is equally effective under less trying circumstances. The richness of Beidelman's approach is that it offers a compelling alternative to anthropology's long-standing interest in normativity, and to bioethics' reductionism, by probing the imaginative dimensions of morality-in-the-making.

Following Beidelman's lead, my project gravitates not to the center but to the boundaries or tentative zones of science, where experimental ideas, products, and associated values proliferate. In the spirit of Michael Lambek's work, too, I am most concerned with that which he terms "ordinary ethics" (2010, 1–36), or those moral processes ubiquitous in daily life yet all too often unmarked as such because of their quotidian nature (see Brodwin 2013).[8] As Lambek explains, "the ordinary is intrinsically ethical and ethics intrinsically ordinary" (3). This is precisely why ethnography is so essential, because it "supplies case material that speaks to the urgency and immediacy yet ordinariness of the ethical" (4).[9] My project differs, however, from Lambek's broadest goals in that I deliberately probe domains that are clearly in flux (an approach, I admit, that can render an investigation both exciting and disorienting). Because moral framing has yet to be "routinized" (again, see Koenig 1988), the ground is never solid in experimental contexts, where potentially no two scientists imagine the value or virtue of animals, human bodies, or experimental products in precisely the same way (see Mol 2002). Experimental domains such as xeno and bioengineering enable pronounced levels of "freedom" of thought (Laidlaw 2002) or, as laboratory scientists themselves like to say, opportunities to "think outside the box." Under such conditions, it becomes possible to track morality-in-the-making in science, where the values that emerge inform the thoughts and actions of a spectrum of scientists focused on a distant—and frequently idealized—future where organ scarcity and human suffering become obsolete.

THE MORAL LOGIC OF EXPERIMENTAL SCIENCE

Organ transplantation is a strange domain in that it requires the excision of presumably healthy parts from the living or the dead so that they may then be transferred to the bodies of seriously ill patients. Transplant's uncanny nature informs widely expressed sentiments regarding its miraculous qualities: surgeons are frequently described as "miracle workers"; the kin of deceased donors imagine their loved ones "living on" in others; living donors speak of a newly forged intimacy with those whose bodies now house their transferred parts; and organ recipients often describe post-surgical life as a "rebirth," a "second chance," or a "second lease on life," turns of phrase that signal how blessed they are to have escaped otherwise terrible fates (Sharp 2006b).

These sorts of sentiments define the more visible aspects of the complex moral realm that circumscribes organ transfer in the United States and, increasingly, abroad. As I describe in detail elsewhere (Sharp 2001, 2002b, 2006b), sentiments and associated behaviors within organ transfer are guided by a set of ideological principles regarding the social values assigned to presumably noncommodified body parts, the transformative experiences associated with the embodiment of organs derived from the living and the dead, the naturalness of such transfers, and anxieties that focus on ever-increasing shortages of what are understood as reusable body parts (Sharp 2006b, 7-24). Organ transfer is rife with official rhetoric that celebrates organ donations as the extraordinary acts of altruistic strangers, organs themselves as gifts that require no reciprocation, and transplant surgery as a medical procedure whose prowess overshadows its short- and long-term economic, clinical, and social consequences. The paradoxical nature of this sociomedical realm is evident in the fact that these highly standardized principles can effectively silence competing or subversive sentiments, including shared desires among recipients and the kin of deceased organ donors to seek out one another; the all-too-frequent lifetime suffering of patients who struggle with the physiological effects and financial burdens associated with daily doses of exorbitantly expensive and potentially toxic immunosuppressants; and widespread social ambivalence regarding clinically orchestrated forms of death, the surgical violation of the integrity of donors' bodies, and the eerie sense that transplant survivors' lives have been saved, extended, or enhanced with fleshy parts acquired from the dead (Sharp 2006b, 25-27).

Set against these disquieting concerns stand the bold alternatives of xeno and bioengineering, two fields that simultaneously embrace the legitimacy of organ transfer while offering alternative solutions that could effectively nullify a range of social obstacles. Whereas scientists working within these two domains may be unaware of the full range of social anxieties outlined above, their work is driven nevertheless by a profound sense of the suffering endured by patients awaiting organs that may never materialize, a scarcity understood as a significant cause of widespread, unwarranted deaths that result from organ failure. This is readily evident, for instance, in the pronounced focus on pediatric needs, where sickly young children and infants might figure prominently in PowerPoint presentations outlining recent experimental advancements. Other presentations underscore opportunities for patients with refashioned bodies to return to their families, workplace, and other hobbies and passions if and when experimental breakthroughs occur. These two experimental domains are rife with hope, possibility, and promise. Because they circumvent the current reliance on parts of human origin, they are also imagined as eliminating the wide spectrum of ethical dilemmas that currently plague transplant medicine, such as how most fairly to distribute scarce resources. In short, xenotransplants and artificial organ design are understood as wiping the moral slate clean.

Such is the surface logic of experimental transplant science, one that frames current endeavors as intrinsically virtuous. Laced throughout both domains is the widespread sense of awe and wonder, or their "what if" promissory qualities. Involved scientists are captivated by the possibilities embodied in simians and pigs (as source animals in xeno), alongside calves and ewes (as test subjects for mechanical organs), and the level of human ingenuity capable of redesigning organs as complex as the heart, lung, liver, pancreas, and kidney. Such sentiments extend beyond the laboratory's walls, too: both xeno and bioengineering are featured widely in the press because of the alternative futures each heralds for transplantation. Bioethicists have repeatedly probed the disquieting social consequences of each, although xeno receives far more attention than do mechanical implants (an issue I return to below) (see Archer and McLellan 2002; Birmingham 1999; Caplan 1992; Donnelley 1999; Faulkner and Kent 2001; Gil 1989; Gorovitz 1987; Koechlin 1996; NCB 1996; Schlaudraff 1999). Yet bioethicists' concerns are frequently bracketed out from scientists' discussions, sentiments among the latter more readily foregrounding human ingenuity as the key to overcoming the potential dangers associated with their respective projects. My overall goal is to probe beneath this seemingly impenetrable layer in an effort to reveal the complex, and often troubled, deeper moral logic that informs these extraordinary experimental efforts.

Within these contexts, Latour's (1999) notion of the "circulating reference" proves helpful as a means to foreground concepts shared across disciplines yet whose polyvalent qualities emerge when scientists must cooperate to settle troubling questions. Whereas Latour's example tracks how specialists apply knowledge and tools from disparate fields to identify where, precisely, a Brazilian forest ends and a savannah begins, I strive to uncover those moments of disjunction, often anchored to specific "boundary objects" (Star and Grieseman 1999), that inspire moral thinking among researchers generally confined to laboratories. Of special significance within experimental transplant research are animal and human subjects, genetically altered creatures, devices of human design, and the human body itself. As I will demonstrate in the final pages of this chapter, specialized moral concerns reference the body's integrity, the sociomoral value of hybrid forms, the meaning of suffering, and the temporal qualities assigned to experimental work.

Body Logic

In *De humani corporis fabrica* (On the Fabric of the Human Body) by the Renaissance anatomist Andreas Vesalius (1973, originally published in 1543), one encounters an array of human bodies. One well-known image depicts a cadaver undergoing dissection, laid out on a table surrounded by a bustling crowd of onlookers assembled there to witness Vesalius at work as he conducts an autopsy. But Vesalius had grander plans, generating a host of exquisitely rendered drawings of male cadavers. Some images feature flayed bodies, their interiors vulnerable and exposed to the elements, but more often these cadavers have been fully stripped of their skin and, assuming various animated poses, display very particular aspects of human anatomy.[10] One figure is composed of pure musculature and appears to dance before a bucolic landscape, its arms reaching out and skyward (figure 1); another consists of a skeleton leaning on a pedestal to contemplate another human's skull (figure 2). Still others include flayed bodies of pure muscle assuming various upright postures, or composed exclusively of a network of nerves that retains the shape of a man standing erect while appearing to float in mid-air. Each of Vesalius's illustrations enables the viewer to imagine radically different sorts of bodies: the human as all bone, muscle, or nerve fiber.

Vesalius proves instructive for revealing the various ways the human body is imagined in contemporary transplant science as well. Not unlike the images in *De humani corporis fabrica*, within transplant medicine one encounters a body that is an anatomical entity, composed solely of its interior. It, too, can be partitioned in radical ways yet remains in some profound sense whole—even when it lacks essential parts—and vital, even though it is made from that which is now dead. In turn, transplantation would remain impossible if vital organs could not be excised, if human parts were not con-

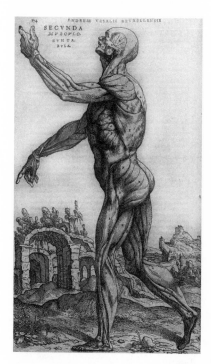

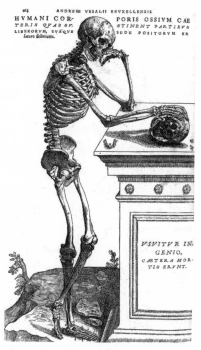

Figure 1. Illustration of human musculature (male figure) from *De humani corporis fabrica* by Andreas Vesalius, Padua, Italy, 1543. (Photo courtesy of the U.S. National Library of Medicine, www.nlm.nih. gov/hmd/ihm.)

Figure 2. Illustration of the human skeleton from *De humani corporis fabrica* by Andreas Vesalius, Padua, Italy, 1543. (Photo courtesy of the U.S. National Library of Medicine, www.nlm.nih.gov/hmd/ihm.)

ceived of as interchangeable, and if replacement parts could not be derived from the dead. These sorts of possibilities emerge because surgery makes it so and because there is widespread social support for such practices. To summarize, the body within the medical domain of organ transfer is fragmented, malleable, interchangeable, and understood primarily by its interior. These principles readily inform efforts within xeno and bioengineering as well. In fact, they are so pervasive as to be taken as unmarked givens in these two experimental domains.

Just as transplant science is actively engaged in the remaking of the human form, related experimental efforts are intent on reimagining the body and refashioning it in still more radical ways. Crucial here is the understanding that the body itself is simultaneously malleable and mutable. Within xeno science, for instance, whereas social activists may consider efforts to fabricate genetic hybrids as monstrous, such an approach is fully naturalized within the field itself. It is, in fact, sensible, realistic, and *moral* to strive to transform humans and/or source animals such that they can be grafted together without incident at the immunological level. Bioengineers understand these principles in yet another way: the human form is inherently flawed, inspiring the efforts of innovative tinkerers who believe that devices of human design could not only replace failing organs but perhaps even surpass the abilities of natal parts. These reimaginings of the human form within xeno and bioengineering offer evidence of beauty, skill, and what we might conceive of as the sublime in experimental science.

In this vein, surgery itself can be seen as a naturalized—and routinized—form of medical tinkering. After all, much of surgery involves opening up the body in order to repair its inner workings and then close it up again. Xeno and bioengineering build upon these established sensibilities, and practitioners within each field understand their efforts as extensions of existing practices. As one physicist colleague said in response to my own reflections on bioengineered organs as a radical innovation, "Yes, but we already do this sort of thing all the time. Look at our kids and our students and [how they use] their electronics—we all need to up our game." Such sentiments—though phrased in different ways—shape core understandings for experimental transplant projects, too.

Hybrid Lives
The body is imagined in radically different ways in xeno and in bioengineering. Xenotransplants insist on the interspecies cohabitation of human and animal within a single organism, where the favored immunological term *chimera* evokes images of the provocative refashioning of patients' bodies. In contrast, bioengineering presents its own sort of blended existence, where mechanical devices are described as "implants" and attempts to "interface" the body with a machine. Nevertheless, both transpecies grafts and artificial devices necessitate embodying parts of nonhuman origin, a technological twinning involving either animal or machine as foretold by Donna Haraway's now classic work, *Simians, Cyborgs, and Women* (1991). Celebrations

akin to Haraway's own regarding radical boundary crossings (between human/animal or human/machine) similarly abound in xeno and bioengineering, where practitioners regularly underscore the liberatory possibilities borne by the remaking of the human and, thus, freeing patients from the crises wrought by organ scarcity.

Whereas members of the lay public, potential patients, social activists, and some bioethicists may be wary of embodying these radical innovations, xeno scientists and engineers view their efforts as part of a long progression within medicine (and science more broadly) to alter the body by extending, enhancing, and saving lives. One need only consider porcine and bovine heart valves, cochlear implants, hip replacements, and animal-derived hormones to realize the extent to which our bodies are indeed hybrid. Some go so far with such now-ubiquitous practices as the use of electronic devices (ranging from smart phones and lap tops to pacemakers and defibulators) as evidence of how frequently our bodies are hooked up or "jacked in" (Gibson 1984) to a range of technologies. In short, in many quarters the post-millennial body is already a hybridized one because we already willingly interface with all sorts of devices such that our bodies are not our own or exclusively us. The naturalization of the newly fabricated self likewise informs futuristic desires in xeno and bioengineering.

Yet that which is deemed most natural generates predicaments, too. As I shall demonstrate in chapter 2, xeno scientists celebrate the monstrous coupling of humans and animals as a desired state of being, boldly exemplified by what today is widely referenced as the chimeric, "humanized" pig. Such constructs destabilize lay understandings of the body's integrity. Xeno scientists are still dogged by troubled histories of earlier, mid-century efforts to implant organs from chimpanzees and baboons into humans, experiments that racialized the boundary of humanness while testing the limits of interspeciality (Sharp 2006a, 2011a, 2011c). Though rarely articulated openly, such efforts mark a deeply troubled moral terrain. Bioengineering faces its own moral challenges, most evident in the denial that inert parts of human design generate any ethical concerns at all (a point I explore in chapter 3). In sum, hybridity exposes moral dangers on multiple fronts, where the starting point flags significant questions about the boundaries of the human body, the importance of guarding its natal integrity, and what in fact qualifies as the "natural" in these experimental pursuits.

Invisible Bodies and the Erasure of Suffering

Amid these celebratory moments is the disquieting effect of the body's erasure. By this I mean not that the physical, tangible aspects of the body escape detection in xeno or bioengineering but, rather, that its subjective properties do. In his work on the "extrahuman world" and the human/machine interface, Michael Jackson (2002, 336) explains that, whereas technologies may seem at times inseparable from us, at others they are uncompromisingly alien. Within the two experimental realms central to my own project, oddly it is not individual bodies and lives that are at stake; rather, it is broadly defined *categories* of bodies (and persons) that suffer—such as dying patients, or those on waiting lists. Also, within experimental clinical and lab contexts, both human and animal bodies are regularly reconfigured as generic entities, where virtually any body, or any animal within a species, can stand in for all others of its kind. This is readily evident in images designed to illustrate the placement of a pig's heart or liver within the body of an experimental subject, or the internal workings of a heart pump and its associated drivelines, and how these are best implanted in a chest and abdomen. Moreover, although lab personnel may give experimental animals pet or personalized names (especially if they are large mammals), when spoken of in professional contexts they remain nameless and numbered (such as "Baboon #17") or otherwise coded (by date of birth, cage or pen position, or original breeding colony, for example).[11] Also, certain creatures fit more comfortably with the scientific imaginary than others: whereas dogs were employed in heart device experiments three decades ago, current researchers prefer farm livestock, often regarding past reliance on canine subjects alongside other domesticated household companions as inhumane. Xeno's own history demonstrates, too, that it has long favored chimps and baboons as ideal human matches, only to shift its desires to the promises embodied in the pig as representative of a newly prized source or "donor" species.

The human body in turn is confined to highly specific parameters. Both fields test their wares on what are typically the most vulnerable subjects. Sometimes these are bioethically suspect choices, such as adult African-

Americans or patients infected with HIV/AIDS or hepatitis C; at other times, they are those most worthy of salvation and thus extraordinary heroics, such as babies and young children (Sharp 2006a, 2011a). Parts, too, are generic: devices come in a limited range of sizes, and fleshy organs are described as if all livers or hearts or lungs universally possess the same dimensions and mass. These extreme forms of reductionism mute more troubling discussions of the moral value of experimentation, where people, animals, and parts are regularly standardized (Sharp 2011b). Furthermore, this is all too often a classless and gender-free world. There is no room (or necessity) for discussions of inequality, whether in reference to something as basic as organ or body size, or as framed by socially significant variables such as race or age or religious faith.

As Jackson (2002) underscores, arguments that celebrate the human/technological interface "seldom take into account the numerous contexts in which doubt, anxiety, or powerlessness tend to make people dread such erasures of the line between themselves and others, or themselves and machines" (336). This erasure of discrete bodies and associated subjective experiences facilitates the erasure of patient suffering, too. In at least one sense, bioethical guidelines are culpable: if one adheres to the four-principle approach, then from the start one justifies extraordinarily invasive procedures through the application of rigorous methods for acquiring informed consent (from humans, at least), and the implementation of protective measures (from anesthesia and analgesics for surgical subjects, to housing facilities, exercise, and cognitive stimulation for animals). As I describe elsewhere (Sharp 2009), I have encountered the uncanny assertion that human suffering does not exist as long as clinical staff respond immediately to patients' reports of physical pain. Yet as revealed through the joint effort of photographer Tim Wainwright and sound artist John Wynne (2008) to document VAD implantees' hospital experiences, those patients' quotidian efforts to cope with post-surgical life impose significant burdens and struggles. Some report unusual existential crises, and among the most striking involve frustrating attempts to forget, drown out, or transform the incessant noise emitted by an implanted heart pump,[12] processes that fall into what Jackson references as "the intersubjective imaginary" (338; see also Rice 2003; Wainwright and Wynne 2008).

What, then, are we to make of psychic pain or existential suffering associated with inhabiting a body powered by non-natal parts? Whereas scientists' futuristic visions may inspire celebration, a patient who consents to a pig liver or mechanical heart implant, even in the short run, must confront the potentially deeply troubling sense that they are no longer fully human. As Jackson underscores, if deep anxiety and ambivalence affect allograft recipients, the sense of alienation is "undoubtedly exacerbated in cases of xenotransplantation" and mechanical implants, too (338–39; see also Lundin 1999; Lundin and Idvall 2003; Papagaroufali 1996, 1997). This is where moral crises of subjectivity ensue. For experimental patients and their kin, it is simply not enough to say that their willingness to undergo such hardships is justified because currently radical efforts could one day transform into routine procedures that save myriad lives. As long as the patient is viewed as a generic body, more complex understandings of experimentation's moral parameters will be denied or silenced; at the very least, the generic body undermines opportunities to explore intriguingly paradoxical—and nascent—social sentiments about hybrid lives.

Animal Biocapital

Just as subjectivity is overshadowed by the generics of the human form, generics is also part and parcel of laboratory animal management, as demonstrated on multiple fronts. For one, a single member of a species must stand in for all others of its kind; moreover, one animal can be replaced by yet another if it falls ill, dies, or is sacrificed; and laboratory animals by definition stand in as generic proxies for humans as a means to test high-risk procedures. Thus, animals are simultaneously expendable and extraordinarily valuable. Indeed, they are specialized specimens: though researchers and lab technicians alike may form strong emotional bonds with particular animals (Sharp 2012), these commodified creatures define lucrative forms of "animal capital," figuring within what Nicole Shukin (2009) labels the "carnal traffic in animal substances" (7). According to Shukin, in such contexts the species divide is "a strategically ambivalent rather than absolute line, allowing for the contradictory power to both dissolve and reinscribe borders between humans and animals" (11). As will become clear in subsequent chapters, the "question of the animal" (11) in experimental transplant science hinges simultaneously on shifting ideas of interspecies proximity or kindredness,[13] the biovalue of one species over others, and the capital gains and, thus, promissory qualities shouldered by one animal versus another. The values assigned to animals, and the morality of their use within science, shift according to the research domain as well as over time when the utilitarian values assigned to certain species enable them to straddle both farm and pharma production. Furthermore, if animals stand in for humans, or if by their mere presence in the laboratory they blur interspecies boundaries, one must also ask, what of human bodies? How, too, might they define a new form of biocapital (Sunder Rajan 2006) when individuals consent to life-endangering experimental procedures (see Abadie 2010) in hopes not only of extending their own lives but also, by giving of themselves (and their bodies), of assisting science in saving others farther down the road?

Promissory Notes

Whereas participation in radical experiments is quite literally a short-lived experience for consenting human (and nonconsenting animal) subjects, the *longue durée* defines a "field of hope" (Rose 2007, 6, after Franklin 1997). According to Rose, "Hope plays a fundamental yet ambiguous role in contemporary somatic ethics" (135),[14] and in such contexts "hope technologies" (Franklin 1997) may figure prominently. As Rose explains, "within such technologies, professional aspirations, commercial ambitions, and personal desires are intertwined and reshaped around a biosocial telos" where "the maintenance of hope has become a crucial element . . . [in the] care for patients with . . . life-threatening illnesses" (135). Although Rose's key example involves nursing care administered to cancer patients (see also DelVecchio Good 2001, 2007), the same is unquestionably true where patients await transplants. Under such conditions, "biology has become imbued with dreams of technological reformation," and the quest "to 'reverse engineer' the condition [of suffering] and then to rectify the anomaly or compensate for the missing elements" is evident in deliberate efforts to reshape life, where "biology is not destiny" (Rose 2007, 51) but, rather, malleable through acts of scientific prowess (or, as opponents assert, of scientific hubris).

In this light, the transplant imaginary is driven by widespread hopes that accompany futuristic medical pursuits. It is this promissory quality of highly experimental work that both facilitates the erasure of (or, at the very least, muted) accounts of subjective suffering and enables involved scientists to pursue research that may never reach fruition in their own lifetimes. The risks, failures, and longing that fuel experimental transplants ride on a host of "probable futures" (Rose 2007, 70), where each potential outcome informs different moral considerations regarding the virtuousness of various experimental paths. As Lambek (2010) similarly reminds us, "ordinary ethics recognizes human finitude but also hope" (4). A final question for me, then, is what sorts of moral promises emerge under the not-so-ordinary circumstances of experimental research, when a project's endpoint rests not in the near present but on a very distant—and perhaps even unattainable—horizon (Guyer 2007; Sharp 2011c)?

THE RECONFIGURED BODY AND THE POLITICS OF HOPE

In a 2012 *New York Times* article, Andrew Cameron, the surgical director of liver transplantation at Johns Hopkins Hospital, reportedly insisted that "people who died for want of an organ did so mostly because there were not enough donors, not because of any shortcomings in medical technology. [Through efforts to encourage Facebook users to proclaim their donor status] 'The math will radically change, and we may well eliminate the problem'" (Richtel and Sack 2012). The calculus of organ scarcity, paired with widespread recognition of patients' undue suffering, nevertheless persists, engendering relentless fear and helplessness among those who vigilantly await news of donated matching organs. Among clinicians, kin, and researchers (all of whom must bear witness to the senseless deaths of patients caught up in the sluggish movement of local, regional, and national waiting lists), even highly experimental—and, thus, life threatening—alternatives assuage their fears by inspiring hope. The very technologies Cameron considers blameless are regarded by many others as inadequately innovative, and likewise they see transplant medicine as desperately in need of far more radical interventions if human lives are to be spared.

The latter configuration of the politics of hope rests heavily on the promissory qualities of "technological reformation" or efforts to "reverse engineer" human suffering (again, see Rose 2007, 51) through experimental efforts to overcome the diseased or flawed aspects of human bodies. Within the transplant imaginary, patients shed personalized medical histories and are devoid of dense networks of kin and friends. That is, within the paired realms of xeno science and bioengineering, subjective experience vanishes, rendering individual suffering invisible. Patients' bodies are abstracted, supplanted by generic categories of affliction framed in turn by the effects of cardiac disease, pulmonary failure, or insulin or dialysis dependence. One also encounters such radical alternatives as primates and "humanized" pigs bred for altogether different forms of human use and consumption, and a host of other astounding, miniaturized gadgetry designed not simply to augment or replace ailing human parts but to outpace their abilities and usefulness. Without question, the transplant imaginary is intently focused on the remaking of the human form, where radical experimentation is framed as an inherently moral pursuit.

Moral thinking in experimental transplant science is driven only in part, however, by "if only" statements or a "what if" line of questioning. The promissory nature of radical body tinkering also exposes competing anxieties about body integrity, the malleability of the human form, the limits of suffering, and the sociomedical dangers of embodied hybridity. In public domains, xeno scientists and bioengineers regularly celebrate the liberatory possibilities borne by their efforts to refashion diseased bodies. Yet the "ordinary ethics" of radical experimentation raises still other disquieting questions regarding experimental prospects. For instance, what are (or should be) the limits of body tinkering? Where does the boundary lie between human and animal vulnerability? What are the social consequences of surgically enhanced hybridity? Highly experimental science does indeed instill heightened moral alertness. In response, ethnographic investigation facilitates the tracking of scientific morality-in-the-making (see Banner forthcoming) and not simply at the center but at the boundaries—or in those tentative zones—where experimental ideas, products, and associated values proliferate. As I demonstrate in the following two chapters, by tracking the "ordinary ethics" intrinsic to laboratory life, one encounters richly textured moral worlds inhabited by scientists who reimagine, reconfigure, and remake the human form.

CHAPTER TWO

Hybrid Bodies and Animal Science

The Promises of Interspecies Proximity

"What am I, as against the world?" "Where is the edge of me?"

Edmund Leach (1964)[1]

From a lay perspective, xenotransplantation is a most peculiar science. Built on the premise that scientific ingenuity could one day overcome the complexities of the human immune system such that our bodies might perceive foreign, animal-derived tissue as "self" rather than "other," this highly experimental domain is driven by desires to accomplish embodied, interspecies hybridity in hopes of alleviating suffering and extending human life. Endeavors to repair the broken bodies of often terminally ill patients are viewed as inherently moral—even heroic—goals within xeno research. Implantable parts range from those derived at the molecular level to whole, fleshy organs, where xenografting could well include the interspecies transfer of pancreatic islet cells, skin grafts, and cardiac valves as well as kidneys, livers, lungs, and hearts. For over a century, xeno researchers have employed a range of what they currently reference as "donor" or "source" animals in experimental contexts. Whereas, in the early twentieth century, cats, dogs, mice, and rabbits dominated experiments, by mid-century other animals rose to prominence, namely primates (most notably chimpanzees and baboons) and, more recently, pigs, each touted at various times as ideal matches for human bodies. Such species preferences—especially where simian and porcine sources are involved—are engendered by scientific desires and other sentiments about the particularities of human/animal proximity.

Animals are understood more generally in science as biological creatures, yet they also inspire complex moral responses. Within xeno specifically, the magnitude of moral thinking is inescapably affected by the broader social values assigned to various species, by the size and function of the parts harvested from them, and by the personal histories of patients whose lives they might one day save, should the match prove immunologically viable. Apes and monkeys usually garner more pity than do pigs; the use of an animal's heart may stir stronger emotional responses than, say, skin grafts, hormones, or islet cells; and pediatric patients are deemed worthy of greater sacrifices than are adults at either the prime or end of their lives. Equally compelling are the more visceral reactions expressed by potential patients[2] and, even more intriguing, by xeno scientists themselves when they are asked to imagine the consequences of having fleshy animal parts implanted within their own bodies.

An understanding that drives this chapter is that, within xeno science itself, the futuristic longing associated with certain types of animals inspires moral speculation, concern, and debate about ever evolving ideas about human/animal proximity. The symbolic weight borne by a particular species—or even just its body parts—informs discussions of xeno's sociomoral worth both within and beyond the laboratory. Animal/human proximity in its most rudimentary form is often framed by notions of kindredness (Franklin 2003, 2007; Taussig 2004). I have written extensively on certain aspects of this theme (Sharp 2006b, 206–41; Sharp 2007, 77–105; Sharp 2011a), and so I touch on it only briefly here. The kindred qualities we assign to chimps, long understood as our close evolutionary "cousins," regularly surface in the ways xeno scientists articulate how and why these and other nonhuman primates[3] define ideal matches for animal-to-human organ transfers. Although such reasoning might well be viewed as a scientific fact, competing arguments espoused by still others about pigs reveal the pronounced efforts involved in legitimating deliberate attempts at hybridity as a form of transspecies kinship. Of special concern to me here, though, is how proximity itself may be approached as a moral category in xeno, and how this is informed specifically by the broader scientific use of animals. The theme of interspecies proximity is important in a field that puts animals to medical use, especially when its proponents are faced with claims in other quarters that various creatures are deserving of special attention because they are endangered and/or highly intelligent.[4] In this light, xeno scientists have most certainly found it necessary to formulate moral positions with care by embarking on what Celia Lowe (2004) describes within the context of species conservation as the "making of [the] monkey" for science. This "making" of animals appears even more deliberate where pigs are concerned. Xeno now strives to remake or refashion (or, perhaps even better put, "render") pigs so that they may be reimagined as even superior to simians as matches for humans.

Apes and monkeys figured prominently in ongoing attempts at transspecies grafting between the mid-1960s and the mid-1990s,[5] a period now often celebrated as a golden era of bold surgical efforts (Sharp 2011c). The broader politics of using such highly sentient creatures, however, subsequently led xeno experts to settle on the pig as the most promising alternative,[6] an approach originally posited by Sir Roy Calne, a leading transplant expert from the United Kingdom (Deschamps et al. 2005, 97; Calne, personal communication, 2010). Because my previous work on allotransplantation began formally in 1991, and this current project in 2004, my research has coincided with what might be thought of as the age of the pig.[7] Nevertheless, when in the company of xeno experts, I regularly bear witness to lively discussions about the comparative values assigned to primates and pigs. Whereas primate proximity rests squarely on evolutionary thinking about species kindredness (Sharp 2011a), arguments that favor pigs are driven by the malleability of porcine anatomy and physiology in the genomic age of science.

Pigs already lay claim to a longstanding history of medical involvement, serving as source animals for porcine-derived insulin, heparin, sinews, guts, skin, and heart valves. As xeno and other animal husbandry experts regularly explain to me, pigs are very similar anatomically to humans (and this is why, for instance, they are employed in biology classes throughout the United States to teach physiology to students).[8] Pigs are also understood as exceptionally hardy and relatively easy to breed and raise for experimental use. They reach reproductive maturity within six to ten months (whereas chimps require several years); a breed sow can produce multiple litters of many piglets over the course of a single year (whereas a chimp's gestational period is eight to nine months and, typically, it has one or at most two off-spring at a time); and pigs can be bred selectively for particular traits that will manifest rapidly within only a few generations. Also, because pigs are classified as neither *endangered* (as are chimps) nor as *laboratory* (as are all primates, alongside rats and other rodents) but as *farm* animals (like the calves, sheep, and goats used by bioengineers who design mechanical organs [see chapter 3]), xeno's use of pigs may seem at first blush to be relatively unproblematic. As I will demonstrate, however, both primates and pigs inspire moral thinking within xeno science, yet very different arguments surround the ways experts imagine and legitimate their use.

Throughout this chapter, I am most concerned with how the experimental value of "source" or "donor" animals is framed in moral terms in xeno science. To be more precise, by "moral" I mean those moments when ambivalence about the scientific and social worth of xeno surfaces. At times, moral quandaries arise in direct response to challenges mounted outside the confines of the laboratory. Such incidents are far more common and acute in xeno science than they are in bioengineering: in the simplest terms, xeno has inspired intensely heartfelt and even belligerent responses from animal activists who regard the work as "mad" or "monster" science. In contrast, the efforts of bioengineers (see chapter 3) are widely regarded, in the words of one inventor, as "ethics free" because they involve the implantation of inert, manufactured devices and not fleshy parts excised from sacrificed animals. This distinction, as we shall see, is overly simplistic, but it does serve to underscore the varied ways in which xeno specialists versus bioengineers must face (and convince) a broader public of the merits of their work. In this current chapter, then, moral domains are circumscribed by the use (or, as challengers put it, abuse) of lab animals. Key concerns for me are how xeno scientists think about animals and what moral sentiments play out in their determination to generate successful forms of interspecies hybridity.

In light of these efforts, I extend the analysis beyond a mere comparative discussion of the social importance assigned to primates versus pigs (see Sharp 2011a, 2011c). I am most interested in how the use of animals more broadly in science affects the moral parameters of the scientific imagination within xeno itself. As such, I decipher how particular species shape the logic of and, ultimately, legitimate embodied hybridity. I draw on ethnographic data generated from my own research, pausing to consider three pivotal moments where the blurring of boundaries between animals and humans present moral quandaries for xeno experts about interspecies proximity. The first pivotal moment centers on a crisis that developed in the United Kingdom (but was certainly possible elsewhere) when a single lab responded to pressure from venture capital that drove it to deplete primate sources at home and abroad, its downfall linked to fiscal insecurity paired with the intensification of animal activism directed specifically at xeno. The second pivotal moment involves the rise of international scrutiny of zoonotic infections in humans, where porcine endogenous retroviruses (PERVs) emerge as a site of special concern within xeno. The third pivotal moment arose during an international conference when leading experts were asked publicly to proclaim whether they themselves would undergo xeno surgeries.

In an effort to organize this somewhat complex discussion, this chapter is informed by three premises. First, if we are to understand how and why xeno experts make use of certain kinds of animals, we must step back and explore the larger and deeply entrenched scientific practice of animal use in the laboratory. I offer this caveat, however: it is not my purpose to map a history of lab animals per se (but see Blum 1994; Haraway 1997; Raines 1991). Instead, I advocate that the widespread use of animals in science more broadly shapes the specifics of moral thinking among contemporary xeno specialists regarding preferences for primates and, now, pigs (see, for instance, Blum 1994; Svendsen and Koch forthcoming). That is, animals of all kinds have been employed within laboratories for quite some time, and associated practices in and beyond the laboratory provide a moral baseline for xeno.

The second premise of this chapter is that the importance of lab animals lies in the fact that they serve as proxies for other things. Most notably, *they approximate nature,* in that a genetically modified lab rat is still, in some sense, a true rat; yet this same creature must also stand in for something radically different, namely humans who may suffer from similar genetic mutations or illnesses, or who must undergo the same medical procedures. In this light, I argue that scientists in many fields constantly engage in the *remaking of nature,* and this in and of itself is understood as a natural scientific—if not more broadly human—trait. A widespread understanding certainly among xeno scientists (if not in other fields, too) is that deliberate efforts to transform an animal's nature epitomize scientific ingenuity, regardless of the discipline. Science, in effect, *re*naturalizes animals to suit its needs, and, further, such efforts are *inherently natural* because they are *inherently human.* Xeno science is deeply informed by this ethos, although xeno proposes among the most radical attempts to alter nature by virtue of its dedication to embodied forms of interspeciality.

The third and final premise is that the remaking of nature as a "natural" process is, nevertheless, a troublesome position. This bold assumption is challenged regularly from outside xeno—and scientific labs more generally—by animal rights and other activists. As my own ethnographic data reveal, at times this same assumption may trouble xeno researchers themselves, especially when they must face the uncontrollable or unforeseen consequences of their work. With data drawn from interactions with xeno experts based in five Anglophone countries (the United States, Canada, the United Kingdom, New Zealand, and Australia), I demonstrate that the richest examples of moral thinking surface when involved scientists must grapple with the illusiveness of the human/animal divide.

Before I advance any further, I must reiterate—as argued in the introduction—that one must not presume that scientists work in isolation, shut away in their laboratories from the everyday world. They are, in fact, deeply integrated within (and are integral to) vast social arenas. Bruno Latour's (1987) idea of "science in action" is especially helpful here, in that laboratory scientists work and thrive within a complex social milieu. "Laboratory life" (Latour and Woolgar 1979), so to speak, is best mapped as a world characterized by simultaneously nested and overlapping domains that extend far beyond a laboratory's walls. Key realms include university or industrial infrastructures, national and international networks of like-minded researchers, complex, heterogeneous populations composed of family and friends, assorted acquaintances and strangers who might be journalists, academics, activists, pet lovers, or potential patients, and, finally, an inquisitive and potentially vast—albeit generally anonymous—reading public (again, see Latour 1987; Latour and Woolgar 1979). In other words, scientists circulate within complicated, intertwined moral worlds, a reality that inevitably leads to challenging and, at times, contradictory understandings (see Mol 2002) of the social importance (or even validity) of their work.

Xeno both typifies science and asserts its own unique moral concerns, the latter marked by a ceaseless dedication to legitimating and promoting ideas about human proximity, first to primates and subsequently to pigs. The overall goal of this chapter is to address how xeno scientists think about the nature of specific kinds of animals, how these animals figure in imaginative, moral understandings of interspeciality as a natural process, and what anxieties surface when they must defend the naturalness of their efforts to blend species within single bodies. The moral principles that guide xeno experimentation are aligned with broader scientific understandings of the human's place in nature (or nature's place in the human world). Guiding premises stand in stark contrast to those espoused by activist opponents, who strive to guard species integrity from deliberate transformative acts within science, and who regard xeno's specific efforts to blend disparate species as inherently unnatural and even monstrous evidence of scientific hubris.

NATURE INTO SCIENCE

Scientists are varied creatures whose interpretations of the meaning, value, or utility of animals are hardly monolithic. One need only consider the range of professions involved in xeno to realize this: dedicated lab researchers include immunologists, geneticists, virologists, large and small animal veterinarians, and, occasionally, transplant surgeons. As a result, an important task here involves differentiating a seeming cacophony of voices in order to decipher patterns in how involved parties think about interspeciality. In an effort to do so, I first address the larger question of how animals are used, and their worth understood, in broader contexts of laboratory work. As we shall see, routinized practices are firmly grounded in the scientific framing of "nature" and, further, in that which is considered "natural" within the laboratory. My efforts to decipher these sentiments require addressing how scientists think of nature's value, how this informs ideas of what is "natural" in science, and, finally, how the notion of "naturalization" (a concept I have pirated from the domain of citizenship) might provide a helpful metaphor for analyzing how science alters or "domesticates" an animal's "natural" qualities to render it useful in the laboratory.

The Human/Animal Divide

Anthropology has long considered its purview the interface of nature and culture. As Philippe Descola and Gísli Pálsson (1996) remind us, the discipline frequently situates the two in a dichotomous and even oppositional relationship (see also Lévi-Strauss 1969; Ortner 1974), where "nature" references "wild" creatures and their habitats, both of which are frequently exploited by humans, a process understood as a distinctive mark of "culture." Humans, in other words, transform natural terrain, fauna, and flora into cultural artifacts. Such transformations may be celebrated as generating, for instance, landscapes of astonishing beauty (as described, for example, by Maurice Bloch [1995] for the Zafimaniry of Madagascar), or they may be condemned as evidence of the destructiveness of our species (as encountered in conservation and ecology literature). In either case, nature, by virtue of its vulnerability, utility, and untamed qualities, contrasts starkly with that which is inherently human.

Within such a framework, the relationship between humans and nature is not an egalitarian one: human societies have always relied on nature for survival and sustenance, often at nature's expense. As our species' history demonstrates, humans regularly exert mastery over nature by clearing forests for fields, fuel, and shelter and by fishing rivers, lakes, and seas or hunting game on land for food, clothing, and medicines and in response to a wide range of other wants and needs. Human adaptability to diverse environments—paired with the domestication of plants and animals—has long been cited within anthropology and beyond as evidence of humankind's civilizing force in the world. Through such processes as culling, harvesting, and domestication, we put nature to work for our survival and sustenance, for ritual purposes, for transport, and even for companionship and as sources of delight.

Animals are widely understood as iconic representatives of nature and, further, of that which is deemed "natural." As such, animals serve as compelling markers of difference, figuring prominently in elaborate, symbolically laden typologies that distinguish the beastly from the civilized (Douglas 1966;

Leach 1964). These typologies may inform pronouncements of who *we* are in contradistinction to that which is *not* human, *not* social, *not* self, *not* I (concepts that are equally central to xeno's logic, applied at the immunological level). Although humans may temporarily assume animal forms (most notably in such religious and ritual contexts as masquerade, possession, dance, dreams, or totemic systems),[9] the key term here is *temporary:* to assume animal qualities without end is a mark of instability or madness, providing poignant evidence that one has lost one's self or one's humanity. Animal typologies, then, are not solely about how we distinguish one creature from another; these same organizing principles inform how we think about ourselves as well. As Edmund Leach (1964) so famously demonstrated, such animal categories as tame or wild, and livestock or pet, inform a complex logic about human-ness. This range of animals, as longtime human familiars, feature prominently in symbolic typologies that correspond with social domains, categories of people, body parts, and religious systems that, in turn, designate domains of human worth, difference, and hierarchy. As Leach explained, "Such classification is a matter of language and culture, not of nature" and, further, "*Our* classification is not only correct, it is morally right and a mark of our superiority" (31, italics in original). In short, animals help humans map the course of moral values within their social worlds; the same may be said for animals in science.

I am most concerned with the meanings assigned to nature as embodied in animals and, more specifically, by those creatures who have been "domesticated," so to speak, for use within a specialized branch of science set on blending humans and animals. With radical forms of xeno hybridity in mind, I ask, first, in what ways are laboratory animals representative of *nature* within scientific contexts? Second, how are particular types of animals understood as *natural* or *unnatural* creations of science by researchers and by other individuals who are based outside the laboratory? Third, what processes—be they scientific or social—make certain species more readily available to scientists, and why are some, but not all, understood as ideal tools for research? That is, what enables scientists more readily to domesticate—or what I will reference as efforts to "naturalize"—certain animals over other species for research purposes? Finally, what are the moral consequences of such processes and associated scientific acts specifically within xeno, where human/animal proximity is of central concern within this field?

Xeno researchers consider attempts to generate sustainable hybrids as natural extensions of scientific prowess in the laboratory. They also understand this work as inherently humanitarian, because they envision saving many lives from suffering in an idealized, distant future (Sharp 2011c). These understandings nevertheless stand in opposition to (and thus push back against) broader social—and, at times, highly politicized and even polarized—sentiments about the moral limits of a scientific discipline determined to blend species. One need only consider the "Weekly Views and News" of the Center for Genetics and Society in Berkeley, California, to encounter an impressive set of online investigative publications generated by the center and other news sources (including *Biopolitical Times*, BBC News, *Forbes Magazine*, *The Independent*, and Reuters) alongside more specific ethical critiques of topics relevant to xeno, under such headings as "animal technologies" and "hybrids and chimeras."[10] Yet no parties have challenged xeno research more fiercely or effectively in recent decades than animal activists concerned with the use and abuse of research animals. The separate domains of xeno science and animal activism delineate a deeply entrenched conflict over moral terrain, where differences might well be irreconcilable because they are built on radically different premises about animal worth, the nature of suffering endured by human and nonhuman research subjects, and the importance of foregrounding human needs. To understand these competing stances necessitates asking broader questions about what, in fact, determines that which is "natural" in the laboratory and the moral premises that drive attempts to conjoin humans with primates or pigs.

Natural Science

In *What Is Nature?* (1995), Kate Soper contends,

> [Nature] is at once both very familiar and extremely elusive: an idea we employ with such ease and regularity that it seems as if we ourselves are privileged with some "natural" access to its intelligibility; but also an idea which most of us know, in some sense, to be so various and comprehensive in its use as to defy our powers of definition. (1)

"Nature" is polysemic with seemingly endless meanings assigned to it, a category that, as Soper explains, includes simultaneously "the totality of non-human matter," "that which is humanly cultivated," "wilderness," and ecological terrains that conceal precious resources. It is, furthermore, "the object of study of the natural and biological sciences" while encompassing "issues in metaphysics concerning the differing modes of being of the natural and the human" (1–2). Nature is thus simultaneously nonhuman, noncultural, yet also part and parcel of our own naturalness. As Soper concludes, "Nature . . . carries an immensely complex and contradictory symbolic load; it is the subject of very contradictory ideologies; and it has been represented in an enormous variety of different ways" (2).

Following Soper's lead, I strive to disentangle the complex and inevitably contradictory understandings of "nature"—and, by extension, that which is "natural" (alongside its inverse, that which is "unnatural" or, as some would contend, monstrous [Rollin 1995; see also Murray 2011]). Like Soper, "my engagement here is essentially with the 'politics' of the idea of nature" (3), but, whereas Soper is most concerned with the vast array of social movements that defend nature, I explore a scientific domain determined to *alter* nature while contending that such a process is itself natural to science. For my purposes, then, "politics" subsumes struggles over meanings and associated social values confined to the rarified realm of xeno science.

In my effort to answer Soper's question "What is nature?" within xeno research, I probe the scientific imaginary as it pertains to the widespread use of and interest in animals. I ask, if nature in its broadest sense is about distinctions and differences that help order human experience and designate that which is *not* human, of what scientific significance are certain kinds of animals, as nature's iconic representatives? Across a range of disciplines—whether anatomy or physiology, evolutionary biology, genetics, or primatology—scientists think comparatively about animals that can be grouped by terrain, morphology, order, or species, or organized hierarchically as vertebrates, mammals, lesser primates, and great apes, where such hierarchies exhibit a telescoped approach that facilitates a determination of animals as our distant versus close evolutionary "cousins" who are still, quite clearly, not us. In so doing, the sciences help us place animals within a continuum stretching from wild to tamed nature, or from wilderness to civilization. When scientists observe wild, captive, or domesticated animals, they do so to learn what they are, what makes them similar to or distinct from us, and what remains unique about our own species.

Oddly, difference and sameness become inseparable, because the closer the association between humans and animals, the greater the possibility that comparative work generates questions, too, of animals' kindredness to us. That is, the farther up one moves within the hierarchy of the animal kingdom, the more like humans certain animals become and, potentially, the greater the possibilities for blurred boundaries. Yet the inverse would also appear to be true: animals that share few human similarities inevitably foreground the specialized qualities and, often (as Leach himself asserted), the superiority of our own species. Xeno science strives to override inter-species difference so as to merge disparate—and, most important, immunologically incompatible—species within single bodies. This drive to create interspecies hybrids is simultaneously a source of significant interest, concern, and anxiety within and beyond the boundaries of xeno experimentation.

The Perplexities of Proximity

Two decades ago, Donna Haraway (1991, 1992) proclaimed that the intermingling of humans and animals in science signals troublesome boundary crossings. Yet she lauded hybrid—and even monstrous—couplings as a liberatory "reinvention of nature," offering humans, alongside—or perhaps best put, *through*—their animal companions, possibilities for reconfiguring gender and class hierarchies. Although Haraway deserves praise for so bold a stance, hers remains at best an unfulfilled utopian vision. Xeno is a science that celebrates the making of "monsters" in the lab, evident in its determination to generate life-sustaining *chimeras,* a term that describes single organisms composed of, or that tolerate, cells of genetically distinct origins. Within xeno labs, the human-like qualities of particular animals render them worthy of lab involvement. Yet scientists who work with lab animals (in xeno and elsewhere) strive quite deliberately to maintain a respectful social distance from animals, foregrounding species difference by regularly evoking morphological and genetic distinctions that are informed by an evolutionary system.[11] In other words, social proximity between humans and animals is tentative at best in research contexts. Even Jane Goodall, very much a champion of primates' dignity and broader rights, provides a poignant example of this. As she has asserted throughout her career, she has always worked alongside chimps as an observer, but she has never sought to live among or as one of them.[12]

In his work on temple macaques in Bali, Agustin Fuentes (2007) demonstrates how primates and humans can "coexist" within the "human niche" (123–24), where monkeys are partially integrated into human practices, a social dynamic that Fuentes labels "sympatry" (126–27). He seeks to answer how humans view, define, perceive, and describe monkeys (and, by extension, other primates) encountered "in-between" or "inside" domains utilized by humans. The interspecies encounters that inevitably occur raise important questions about "nonhuman primates' role in human *place*" (133, italics in original), where social distinctions are nevertheless maintained, as evident when Balinese ideas are contrasted to tourists' sentiments toward monkeys. Whereas Balinese view macaques as food, pets, performers, and figures that populate a religious pantheon, when foreign tourists encounter these animals, they might well view them as "little people," a fleeting social move Fuentes identifies as "theoretical familiarity and pseudokinship" (123–24, 127, 134). As these contrasting responses reveal, specific values assigned to animals then determine the limits of interspecies sociality, where boundaries shift according to context, interactions, and the pragmatic and emotional tenor of human needs.

Within laboratory settings, sympatry takes a radically different turn. Here, interspecies distancing is far more pronounced than that displayed by either Balinese or tourists in response to temple macaques or, if we return once again to Goodall, in her encounters with both wild and captive chimpanzees. Within xeno labs—be they based in the United States, the United Kingdom, Canada, New Zealand, or Australia—proper research procedures mandate practices that insure a respectful social distance is maintained between disparate species. Animals—regardless of whether they are zebra fish, hamsters, rats, pigs, tamarins, baboons, macaques, or chimps—must each be housed in specified types and sizes of enclosures, fed, cleaned, cared for in highly standardized ways, and handled and managed over the course of a twenty-four hour day in ways dictated by university or industrial, state or provincial, and national or even international regulations. Without question, lab-based humans may grow fond of or emotionally attached to certain animals (Sharp 2012); such creatures are, nevertheless, regarded simultaneously as laboratory property and as research tools subject to constant human scrutiny. As such, lab animals are first and foremost highly specialized work objects (Hogle 1995) on whose welfare research is unquestionably dependent,[13] a factor that shapes moral thinking among involved scientists about their value and use.

Under such conditions, encounters with nature in the laboratory require a very different sort of moral framing than that assigned to wild (or, in the case of temple macaques, semi-wild) creatures. Indeed, throughout the course of my research I have regularly encountered widespread human affinity for pigs in laboratories and their associated farms, such that scientists often pose with them, especially if they are still piglets (see figure 3). In one instance, the photo had clearly been shot at home or in a lounge with the piglet resting on the back of a sofa. As lab animals, they most certainly are unlike others that roam freely in open terrain where they eat, mature, defecate, play, mate, forage, and die. Instead, their breeding, selection, and culling for scientific use together define a specialized type of domestication (Raines 1991). Most important, lab animals are always proxies for other things: first, because they approximate nature, albeit under controlled conditions; and, second, because they must approximate, in some form, things human. As such, our relationship to them is reconfigured as a rather unorthodox form of pseudokinship (again, see Fuentes 2007).

Lab animals are therefore unusual creatures, falling somewhere between domesticated stock and prized commodities that perform specialized tasks as unique work objects. In writing specifically of commodities, Igor Kopytoff (1986) distinguishes between those objects that possess unique value or "singularity," set against the "mundane" and "commercialized" (73–84). Interestingly, laboratory animals (who are unquestionably commodified creatures)[14] manifest both qualities as once. We need only consider the lab rat, for example, to realize that it stands in as something larger than itself that marks it simultaneously as singular and generic. As a creature easily replicated and, thus, easily replaced by others bearing the same cell lines, genetic traits, infections, and so forth, a single rat stands in for all rats of its kind. Yet its kind is also valued for the unique promises it bears to mimic highly specific human outcomes in reference to, say, obesity, rheumatoid arthritis, diabetes, lupus, or dementia. These simultaneous yet seemingly

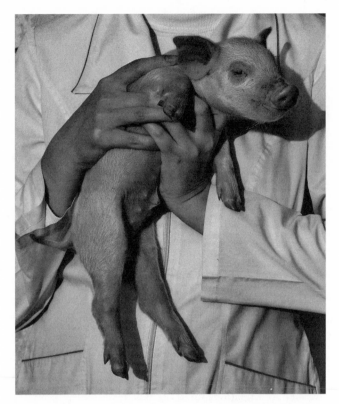

Figure 3. Lab researcher holding a piglet. This photograph circulates widely within xenotransplant circles, employed regularly on web pages and in blogs and PowerPoint presentations (often with the piglet's hind legs cropped out). Visually it promotes the ease at which interspecies proximity—and sociality—may occur, facilitated by the pristine quality of the image and cleanliness of both subjects, the cuteness of the piglet held carefully by the researcher, and the fact that the human's hands are generally read as female (and, by association, caring). When reprinted in color, the pinkness of the pig and the pair of hands enables them to blend into one another, too. ("Pig in Female Hands," photograph by Anatolii Tsekhmister, taken in 2009, iStockphoto #9165598, www.istockphoto.com.)

competing qualities are what render the lab rat so extraordinarily valuable. Such principles also inform xeno research, where the distinct qualities of primates and pigs enhance their value as suitable human proxies (such that one shares evolutionary, the other anatomical, proximity). Each in their own way, to borrow a phrase from Kopytoff, is "symbolically supercharged," falling within a specialized "moral hierarchy" of value (74) where they are perceived or made to be like us but certainly are not the same as us.

The Naturalized Laboratory Animal

Lab science thus transforms a species' wild nature into a newly domesticated utilitarian creation. As a way to unpack this particular type of domestication specifically in the context of xeno research, I employ the concept of "naturalization," borrowed from the language of citizenship, to signal the transformative processes imposed on lab animals. As a process, naturalization is, in a sense, always tentative. This is not because it is a distinct legal status where people, at least, are concerned: in fact, human rights and privileges may be indistinguishable between the naturally born and the naturalized.[15] Naturalization is tentative, nevertheless, in that it requires a deliberate and methodical shift from one status to another and thus retains a history always distinct from that claimed by the "naturally" born. Just as naturalized citizenship requires deliberate efforts to alter the "nature" of individuals, the domestication of animals for laboratory use marks a very particular—and peculiar—form of remaking creatures for science (see Lowe 2004).

In this light, scientific labor ultimately alters the intrinsic value of animals. The naturalized laboratory animal is no longer (and never can be) the same as its truly wild (and thus "purely natural") counterpart, its value resting on its ability to approximate both animal and human life. Because such animals are never truly wild or truly "other" (that is, human), they inspire a host of moral quandaries founded on questions of the animal's integrity. For instance, how representative of its kind is a laboratory chimp when compared to those born and raised in the wild?[16] How porcine is a pig selectively bred specifically to produce organs of human size? As scientifically domesticated creatures, they live under artificial—that is, "not wild" and thus "unnatural"—conditions. This is even more pronounced given that their genetic "nature" may have been so fully altered for experimental purposes as to render them, at a molecular level, partially human.

These lab-based efforts at naturalization are laced nevertheless with subtle, underlying anxieties over what it means to alter an animal species so profoundly. Such anxieties can be pronounced in xeno science, such that transgenic animals are imagined today as promissory creatures (Guyer 2007; Sharp 2011c) caught up in a process of becoming something else that has not yet been fully realized. Whereas naturalized citizens (depending on national and historic contexts) may claim a full suite of rights, they nevertheless remain distinct from (natural) citizens who claim necessary parentage or ancestry. So, too, the lab animal is never fully the same as other wild (or "natural") members of its species. Instead, the lab rat, or rabbit, dog, pig, or chimp, have all been *renaturalized* or *retooled* by science. Such configurations are rife with contingencies, precisely because naturalization as I use it here signifies both a status always in flux and, by extension, one that drives moral thinking that is subject to constant debate or revision.

Whereas, at first blush, interspeciality may seem relatively unproblematic, it does breed a host of sometimes muted, sometimes pronounced anxieties within and beyond the laboratory. Scientists, after all, are not simply socialized by peers to think plainly, clearly, rationally, and in lock step with others about experimental animals. Instead, I contend that anyone who works with lab animals must face questions about the moral boundaries of their use, precisely because they must resolve conflicting personal sentiments in their efforts to remake them for science (Lowe 2004).[17] For instance, researchers might develop deep attachments to individual animals while employing them behaviorally, genetically, or surgically. This is why they can—and must—think of animals simultaneously as unique creatures for whom they feel emotional affinity, as research tools invaluable to their work, and as replaceable (and even expendable) subjects whose value ends (and, often, their lives terminated) once necessary data are amassed.[18] Such sentimental differences may appear irreconcilable, but, when framed by a scientific ethos, they reemerge as complementary aspects of laboratory life. This is what makes animal research a moral project, one anchored by the promise to further human knowledge and, specifically in the medical sciences, to save human lives further down the road. As we shall see, however, even these efforts have their moral limits.

ANIMAL FAMILIARS IN XENO SCIENCE

Xeno science is driven by the determination that the immune system might well be fooled into perceiving foreign tissue as "self" rather than "other," as immunologists explain, yet the field has nevertheless struggled tirelessly to overcome such hurdles. This extraordinary challenge is reflected in the now often quoted words of Sir Roy Calne (2005), a foundational figure in multiple arenas of surgery and research who posed the question, "xenotransplantation—the future of transplantation, and always will be?" Xeno experts assert efforts at human/animal hybridity as a natural propensity of our species, and, as I detail elsewhere (Sharp 2011c), speakers at xeno conferences regularly inflect their talks with references to centaurs, Egyptian and Hindu deities, and a range of other mythological monsters as evidence of hybridity's longstanding cultural and historical antecedents.

Nevertheless, contemporary xeno science extends back only about a century. Among the field's most celebrated founders is Alexis Carrel, a French-trained surgeon awarded the Nobel Prize in 1912 for his accomplishments in vascular surgery. Carrel had a truly experimental mind, demonstrated by the astonishing array of lab activities that marked his career at the Rockefeller Institute for Medical Research in New York City. Carrel's celebrity within and beyond medicine is reflected in the fact that he appeared twice on the cover of *Time* magazine.[19] He was, for instance, the first to perform a coronary artery bypass (the subject was a dog); he developed the first antiseptic (sodium hypochlorite, buffered with sodium bicarbonate); and he attempted still other experiments on heart resuscitation, organ perfusion, skin grafting, the growth of animal and human tissues outside the body, and mouse genetics (the latter making him an early target for animal rights activists). Carrel's xeno research involved experimental kidney transfers among sheep, pigs, goats, dogs, and primates.[20] At a time when the immune system was not well understood, Carrel's xeno experiments ran awry rather quickly, with catastrophic results for the implanted (not to mention the sacrificed source) animal,[21] and, by the end of the first decade of the twentieth century, Carrel had abandoned this research (D. Friedman 2007, 1–16). Contemporary xeno experts nevertheless speak of Carrel with great nostalgia, celebrating him for his bold, anticipatory efforts in the field.

The xenografting of whole organs received only sporadic attention over the next forty years,[22] but its seriousness as a sustained surgical focus involving the transfer of whole organs dates back to the mid-twentieth century. These efforts arose alongside significant strides made in allotransplantation, and in this way it both enabled and shadowed the latter field.[23] Whereas human-to-human organ transfers are now regularly proclaimed as among the greatest miracles of contemporary medicine, xeno has been plagued by both significant immunological failures and social challenges. Although little known outside xeno circles, a number of foundational giants within transplant medicine laid claim to additional expertise in xeno research, in large part because techniques that made human organ transfers successful were frequently informed by knowledge derived from animal experiments (as is true, of course, in many other fields). Several of these surgeons also tried implanting animal grafts in humans, though with little success. Their efforts correspond with two key periods. The first spans the mid-1960s to the mid-1990s, a period often regarded by xeno scientists as a golden (albeit failed) era of high-risk experimentation[24] when several surgeons tried implanting chimps' and baboons' organs in terminally ill patients.[25] The second key period corresponds with the mid-1990s to the present, a time when miniature, hybridized pigs have come to dominate research. Currently, an array of specialists' experiments focus on the cross-species grafting of porcine organs into baboons and macaques in hopes of one day attempting such surgeries in humans.

Tracking the History of Blended Bodies

The broader historical relevance of xeno science to transplant surgery's success is evident, for instance, in the efforts of the renowned surgeon Christiaan Barnard. Although best known for attempting the world's first heart transplant in South Africa in late 1967, Barnard also performed the first kidney transplant in his country only a few months earlier (having practiced necessary surgical techniques on dogs). Throughout his long career, Barnard conducted a host of other transspecies organ transfers involving monkeys and other creatures, and in so doing he trained several specialists now considered the undisputed leaders of xeno research who had come to work in his labs [David Cooper, personal communication, 2009; see also Deschamps et al. 2005).

The logic that informed Barnard's efforts involved testing ideas and techniques on animal species before attempting them on humans, and whereas the primary goal was to implant human organs in ailing patients, several instances were designed specifically to test interspecies proximity. As detailed in my introduction, ever-growing anxieties over sources of human organs now fuel many efforts in transplant research, yet of equal importance has been a more general desire within xeno to circumvent altogether a reliance on human donors. Thus, from the 1960s on, transplant giants such as James Hardy, Claude Hitchcock, Keith Reemtsma, Thomas Starzl, and Denton Cooley all attempted primate-to-human organ transfers (Deschamps et al. 2005).[26] In addition, a relatively unknown example of porcine xenografting was attempted in 1966 by René Kuss, a French urologist who transferred two pig kidneys to a single patient. The graft failed immediately and the patient soon died, even though Kuss removed the organs after forty-eight hours. As Kuss himself reported years later, "I retained from this painful experience a xenophobia for xenografts which remains with me today!" (as reported in Cooper 2007).

As is true of many experimental and high-risk surgeries, attempts at xenografting throughout the 1960s inevitably involved terminally ill and, sometimes, even pediatric (Sharp 2006a) patients, offering special evidence of the urgency to save lives through what were still considered drastic means. Other experimental surgeries occurred in Italy, France, and South Africa (Auchincloss Jr. 1988; Cooper and Lanza 2000; Deschamps et al. 2005), although the United States was by far the most active site for such efforts. As I illustrate elsewhere (Sharp 2011a, 2011c), these highly experimental surgeries offered a testing ground for determining not only human/simian proximity but sometimes more specifically racialized human/simian evolutionary, genetic, and immunological similarities, with numerous high-profile surgeries conducted in the Deep South that all too often involved African-American subjects. Xeno patients typically died within days from such complications as cardiogenic shock, vascular hyperacute rejection, and sepsis. Two notable exceptions were a woman who survived four months with a baboon's liver and another patient who lived for nine months with a chimpanzee's kidney.[27] The more common, dramatic failures meant that another two decades would pass before anyone attempted more surgeries in the United States or elsewhere.

In 1984, with the arrival of the new—and, ultimately, highly effective—immunosuppressant cyclosporine, a relatively unknown surgeon named Leonard Bailey in Loma Linda, California, made a bold attempt at transspecies grafting by implanting a juvenile baboon's heart in an anonymous twelve-day-old infant girl known at the time only as Baby Fae. She survived twenty-eight days before succumbing to the devastating effects of xeno graft rejection. The outrage over Bailey's hubris within transplant circles was pronounced. As I detail elsewhere (Sharp 2011a), Bailey was denounced for his efforts by better known transplant surgeons as well as by many bioethicists. The demise of Baby Fae led to a decade-long, self-imposed moratorium on human xenografting by xeno experts.

This moratorium remained intact nearly universally until 1993,[28] when Thomas Starzl, a leader in kidney and liver transplantation, temporarily revived the field by testing the effectiveness of a new immunosuppressant known as FK506 (*tacrolimus*), implanting baboon livers in two terminally ill adult patients based in Pittsburgh who were infected with HIV and/or hepatitis C and who at that time could not qualify for allografts.[29] Both surgeries proved fatal: one patient survived seventy days; the other remained in a coma until he died twenty-six days later. Although Starzl had obtained approval for a third surgery, he terminated the study when faced with insurmountable immunological hurdles and widespread media coverage that grew increasingly critical over time (Starzl et al. 1993).

By the 1990s, animal activists based in the United States, the United Kingdom, and elsewhere had become increasingly vocal in their outcry against the abuse of laboratory animals, and xeno science was a target for especially virulent protest, as evident in Starzl's case. As ethicist Bernard Rollin asserts in *The Frankenstein Syndrome: Ethical and Social Issues in the Genetic Engineering of Animals* (1995), attempts to alter the intrinsic nature of animals exposed a widespread "denial of ethics" as a guiding ideological principle in science (11). Rollin proffers the field of genetic engineering as evidence that scientists widely ignored risks, their inability to anticipate the unintentional consequences of their work providing evidence of a "syndrome" of sorts that he likens to Dr. Frankenstein's "rampaging monster" (67). Such sentiments were shared by animal activists, who were deeply troubled by what they perceived as medical hubris. For instance, following Starzl's failed attempts at baboon xenografting, he became known in some activist circles as "Dr. Starzlstein" and the field more generally as "Frankenscience."

As in Bailey's case, scrutiny and protest were not limited to the United States. One group that I will call NoXeno[30] emerged first in the United States in the 1990s but soon gained international momentum with outposts in Europe, New Zealand, and Australia. When the added dangers of porcine zoonoses surfaced (see below), NoXeno spearheaded a legal investigation of lab activities in the United States, and among its favored images was a photo of a human face sporting a pig's snout that is still employed widely in the greater activist community, sometimes accompanying an essay entitled "Where will the next plague come from?"[31] NoXeno was part of a larger international contingent of activists who questioned, challenged, and protested xeno scientists' efforts. Xeno scientists in New Zealand and Australia, for instance, report struggles with activists akin to those of their colleagues elsewhere. The United Kingdom offers an especially involved set of circumstances as a country with a long history of anti-vivisection movements as well as significant strides in genomic science.[32] By xeno experts' accounts, they witnessed perhaps the most pronounced and violent struggle over the legitimacy of their use of laboratory animals. As one Australian scientist reflected in 2009, "afterwards, xeno was dead in the water in the U.K."

Today, U.K.-based activists, bioethicists, and scientists alike boast that their nation's legislation is the most rigorous in the world, and many were able to outline extemporaneously during interviews the principles of what are known today as the "Three Rs" and the "Five Freedoms,"[33] regulatory principles that define the core of animal welfare legislation and practice in their country. When asked during interviews to reflect back on the mid-1990s, xeno experts often reported harrowing experiences that involved anonymous death threats, attacks on their homes or those of their colleagues, and laboratory break-ins. Various inquiries ensued: the first effort was sponsored by the Nuffield Council[34] in conjunction with a Working Party,[35] resulting in a comprehensive evaluation of the field (NCB 1996); the second was a nearly simultaneous—and, within Nuffield, an unexpected spinoff—effort through the Department of Health that generated a document now known as *The Kennedy Report* (DOH-UK 1997).[36] Together these served to generate the rather short-lived U.K. Xenotransplantation Interim Regulatory Authority (UKXIRA); it was designed to regulate solid organ xenotransplants but was "quietly disbanded" in 2006 (McLean and Williamson 2007;

see also McLean and Williamson 2005). As one involved member explained to me, by 1993 Nuffield had identified genetic screening, the use of human tissue, and xenotransplantation as issues of key bioethical concern in the United Kingdom, but by 1995 xeno had assumed a special urgency because of ongoing activities that posed potential social dangers.

These diverse events had several important consequences. Both documents had a significant impact on shaping subsequent regulatory approaches to xeno research. As a Nuffield member explained, the bioethics of developing transgenic animals emerged as an early focus of concern, and members reached consensus fairly quickly that "no higher primates—this meant chimps" should be used in research (members were somewhat more tentative about baboons).[37] Today, both documents continue to inform discussions over the ethical treatment of animals and the moral parameters of xeno and related branches of science (McLean and Williamson 2007). In other quarters, several high-profile activists were tried and went to prison; furthermore, as one bioethicist explained, the "fallout" or "expected exchange" was that xeno (and other laboratory) scientists were charged to think more carefully, critically, and deeply about the moral parameters of their work. A subsequent undercover report entitled "Diaries of Despair," produced in 2000 by the animal rights group Uncaged, deepened national antagonism toward xeno research and, I must add, inspired critical reflection among those xeno experts I have interviewed who have read it (Lyons 2000; see also Uncaged 2007). Yet another significant consequence has been the ongoing ban on primate xenotransplants in the United Kingdom (a development mirrored in the other four Anglophone countries where my research is based). The question, then, is how do involved xeno experts reflect back on these events, and how did their involvement shape current moral thinking? In an effort to answer this, I turn to a set of events that took place at a firm I refer to as XenoLife.

Source Animals as Scarce Biocapital

In 1995, XenoLife, a small yet cutting-edge xenotransplant lab based in the United Kingdom, proclaimed promising results. XenoLife was emblematic of a key shift in xeno efforts, working just as the field was transitioning from using primates as donor species (as evident in Starzl's experimental baboon surgeries) to developing hybridized pigs whose genome incorporated human material in hopes of implanting their parts in people. As several xeno researchers stressed during interviews, this shift was largely enabled by efforts based in Scotland that produced Dolly the Sheep, the first mammal to have been successfully cloned from an adult cell.[38] Though still deeply embedded in early experimental attempts to graft pig organs in primates (who now stood in as human proxies of an altogether different sort), Xeno-Life soon faced substantial pressure from its investors, which included a multinational pharmaceutical company, to move rapidly toward human trials. Although tens of millions of British pounds had been invested already in XenoLife, the firm soon found itself on the verge of financial collapse. Xenotransplant surgeries indeed looked promising, yet persistent and complex immunological hurdles signaled a long uphill climb before true hybridity could be attained, and a number of experts based elsewhere believed that such results most likely would not be possible for a long time to come. Venture capital had nevertheless grown impatient for promising results.

Thomas Maeder and Philip Ross (2002), writing on the investment risks involved in nonhuman transplant technologies, demonstrate how fickle venture capital can be and how its desire for profit can push industry to assume a pace that is at odds with the comparative plodding of laboratory experimentation. Experimental success is dependent, after all, on a high tolerance for the rigors of an associated trial-and-error approach. The integrity of the experimental method relies on hypothesis testing, requiring that meticulous attention be given to imagining, designing, and running trials, all of which must be repeated if an experiment fails, necessitating a reformulation of a hypothesis and redesign of procedures, or, if it appears to succeed, in order to confirm through repetition the reliability of data. All ideas, procedures, and processes remain tentative unless they can be replicated successfully in one's own and in others' labs. Experimental life, then, requires extraordinary patience, because successful outcomes may take years, or even a lifetime, to achieve. In stark contrast, venture capital prefers rapid results and thus has a very low threshold of tolerance for what it all too often perceives as the ponderous and even tedious qualities of scientific inquiry. Xeno is an especially frustrating domain in this regard: a surfeit of immunological challenges ensures at best a protracted pace before reliable results emerge.

Within all five countries where I have conducted research, experimental work is heavily dependent on an influx of capital, whether through university investment, federal agencies that target pure science, military sources, pharmaceutical corporations, individual investors, or relatively small non-profits (that, in the case of transplant research, may advocate for patients' needs). The scientists I have encountered in the course of my own work—be they from XenoLife or elsewhere—generally speak of cobbling together funds from multiple sources, and venture capital (most often from private investors and pharmaceutical firms) is identified as that which exerts the greatest pressure to generate quick (and, thus, potentially impossible) results. Work dependent on primates is especially challenging financially in large part because of the regulations that address their welfare and that stipulate the high-cost conditions of their care and subsequent retirement. Within such a climate, XenoLife was faced with the choice of either providing clear evidence of success or going under.

The moral repercussions of these events are reflected in an account offered by Brenda Watson, a veterinarian in her late thirties trained in large animal research who worked for XenoLife in the mid-1990s. As she explained to me during an interview in 2010, XenoLife depended heavily on both pigs as source animals and monkeys as recipients (and, thus, proxies for testing future implantation in humans). In an effort to quell pressure and retain financial support, within a single year XenoLife ran through—and depleted—the entire supply of rhesus macaques available for experimental use within the United Kingdom. It then proceeded to do the same on the Continent, exhausting captive rhesus colonies throughout Western Europe. Faced with the ceaseless pressure from investors to produce rapid results in a field rife with significant immunological challenges, XenoLife then sought desperately to acquire baboons captured in the wild in Kenya and elsewhere in East Africa, a move informed by the assumption that "baboons were mere pests" in these locales (this same phrase was used sardonically by a Nuffield Council member in a later interview).[39] XenoLife's management presumed that wild baboons could prove to be a boon for a science desperate for monkeys.

In the face of such drastic proposals, Watson and several of her colleagues resigned from XenoLife on moral grounds, appalled by ideas she regarded as "horrifyingly neocolonial" in addition to blatantly callous attitudes regarding the "expendability" of animal life. When she was in her early twenties and just beginning her career, she had originally imagined xeno as an exciting lifetime profession; yet after her experiences with Xeno-Life, she charted a different course. As she explained to me, she initially accepted the job because it would enable her to conduct original, transgenic research with rodents and pigs, but she soon found herself involved in primate surgeries as well, which ran contrary to her beliefs regarding the misuse of highly sentient animals in science. She had grown up on a farm, where she learned to respect—and even have a certain awe for—animals. When she was asked to assist in the transport and subsequent lab-based care of wild baboons, she resigned, even though she faced unemployment. Today she cares for laboratory animals of all sorts, a job she finds deeply fulfilling, but she regularly asserts her presence when she believes animals are being "sacrificed" (that is, euthanized) unnecessarily or in large numbers. Jokingly, she said some lab technicians call her "The Guardian Angel" whereas others (generally behind her back) prefer "The Enforcer." She even keeps a range of species at home that she has rescued from laboratories just before they were scheduled to be euthanized. Even though this practice runs contrary to regulations, some lab technicians will approach her when they wish to save the lives of certain, favored creatures.[40]

Brian Carrithers, another former XenoLife employee now in his midforties, is a geneticist with a longstanding interest in swine-based zoonoses. In a 2010 interview, he elaborated on how his moral stance on animal care developed in response to events that unfolded at XenoLife, where he worked until around 2000:

> BC: I was struck by [different approaches among staff involving] the dignity of the animal [set against] the "throwaway" aspects of animals. . . . There was a crescendo of activity [at XenoLife in 1995] to convince the regulatory guard at [the national level and within the investing pharmaceutical firm] . . . to then move on to [human xeno trials]. There was pressure to rattle on [that involved using many animals] in pig-to-primate transplants. . . . [T]hey were doing them in bunches of 10 to 15 every two months [or so].
>
> LS: That's an awful lot.

BC: Yes. Well, [as you've heard,] we [had] depleted the resources of rhesus macaques. . . . We used up *hundreds* . . . I felt I was being used, not as a talent, but as a, hmm, [searches for an appropriate word] . . . if I could give my *blessing,* but increasingly . . . [well, you see, as reported] in "Diaries of Despair" [there were] unnecessary procedures [conducted on animals for xeno research]. . . .

LS: Could you tell me [specifically about the pigs]?

BC: Oh, [we used] *hundreds.* . . .

LS: [later in the interview:] What happened to the animals at that point [when the research ceased and XenoLife closed]?

BC: They were euthanized . . . the semen was stored, the eggs were [harvested and] stored [as well], the germ . . . stored in the U.K. We argued that the pigs were perfectly safe for human consumption, but the government . . . didn't want [to introduce] GM [genetically modified] animals [as sources of food].

LS: How many animals were there [that were euthanized]?

BC: We had a . . . sow breeding unit [in several countries]. . . . A typical sow has two litters a year, so that means around 1,000 offspring per year [in each unit]. [We had] maybe 500 pigs in each [location abroad] and maybe [another] 200 [at XenoLife]. Each [site] would have had 10 [breeding] sows [so the rest were piglets]. I'd say 1,500 animals [were euthanized].

LS: And what about the monkeys? Were they euthanized?

BC: Oh, no. [They were] too valuable. The ones that had not been used in experiments were then [moved to] other research facilities. The ones that had been involved in experiments [were euthanized]. . . . There were often battles between the scientists and the vets [at the labs]. . . . At the endpoint [the vets were told] the animals must be euthanized and the transplanted animals were [euthanized as well].

Today Carrithers's immunological lab work is driven by a determination to develop research protocols focused solely on in vitro research that targets responses at the cellular level. With this approach, he strives to ensure that as few animals as possible are sacrificed in the name of science. Carrithers is deeply devoted to "the Three R's" of animal welfare in laboratory research, and he gave me a detailed account of the meanings of "Replace, Reduce, and Refine" as well as a more cursory overview of the "Five Freedoms." He also works as an instructor at a leading university, where he integrates these moral codes of conduct into his lectures to undergraduates, hoping that his students will form a new vanguard in xeno and other branches of animal research. As he put it, "Better to derive hundreds of samples for research use from a single animal than to expend the lives of hundreds in the name of one experiment. I hope that this can be the future of animal research [in the United Kingdom]."

The Zoonotic Threat

As if grassroots animal activism over the treatment of captive lab animals were not enough, primates and pigs have proved to be uncertain and potentially dangerous choices as source animals. The United Kingdom was on heightened alert for zoonoses that might infect humans, most notably in response to the outbreak of bovine spongiform encephalopathy, or "mad cow disease," in 1996. In 1997, Jonathan Allan, a virologist based in San Antonio, Texas, well known for work that identified the connection between AIDS and HIV, sounded an alarm for xeno when his ongoing research revealed the ease with which primate viruses could infect human tissue. As he proclaimed during an aired discussion on Australian National Radio in 1997, "There is virtually no way to eliminate even the known infectious agents from the baboon. So what we're doing is we're playing Russian roulette in terms of placing viruses into the human population" (ABC 1997; see also Allan 1996). Yet another London-based team, under the direction of virologist Robin Weiss, conducted work on swine diseases and reached conclusions similar to Allan's about the dangers of porcine xenografts (Patience et al. 1997; Weiss 1998a, 1998b). Although monkeys were already held suspect for a host of viruses presumed to have passed from them to humans, pigs suddenly rose to prominence with the discovery that swine herds potentially worldwide harbored endemic (and often symptom-free) infections of porcine endogenous retroviruses (PERVs), essentially the equivalent of HIV in pigs. As the work by Weiss's team demonstrated, PERVs bore the threat of jumping the species barrier if living porcine tissue were to be implanted in human patients' bodies. This meant not only that it might make patients ill but that it could generate an epidemic if such patients were then to infect family, neighbors, coworkers, and strangers.

In response, several prominent scientists broke rank, questioning the legitimacy and safety of xeno research. These experts had grown increasingly concerned by the prospect that zoonoses could wreck havoc in human populations. A pronounced effort was spearheaded by Fritz Bach, a Harvard-based immunologist who called for a moratorium that brought even his own research to an end (Bach 1996; Bach et al. 1998; Bach and Ivinson 2002; Bach et al. 2001; see also Groth 2008; Michaels 1998; Sypniewski et al. 2005). Although animal activists I have interviewed remain skeptical of Bach's intentions (claiming he staged subsequent FDA hearings not in order to stop xeno but to quell protests), his actions were forceful enough to help instigate a ban on implanting porcine grafts in humans in the United States and, one might argue, worldwide. Notably, Bach has yet to resume xenograft research.

Such concerns over zoonotic infections inspired responses elsewhere. As Carrithers explained to me, beginning around 1996 xeno research in the United Kingdom had already shifted to a near-exclusive interest in producing pathogen-free pigs, a process that relied heavily on international networks of xeno experts based elsewhere who took on the task of raising small isolated herds of about ten sows each in Europe, Canada, the United States, and Japan:

BC: [In order to produce] QPF [qualified pathogen free] herds . . . ours were based in Canada. They were kept in a sterile environment, they ate irradiated food, there were strict barriers [that humans had to pass through to prevent the introduction of pathogens], then we'd do an organ harvest. We'd get a human [transplant] surgical team to remove an organ to prove it was possible to harvest a porcine organ pathogen free for human use.[41]

LS: I've heard there really are no pathogen-free pigs, though. Is this true?

BC: [Actually,] we did manage to do this, but the one we couldn't exclude was PERV[s]: and this is what shut down [the project in the end], plus [there remains the problem of] wild caught captive [pigs with] PERV[s]. You see, it's embedded in the genome, it's in the gene line [of pigs. The pigs might not have symptoms but] . . . it could pop out in the tissue . . . and it could unfortunately infect human cells, and it can be oncogenic: they [go back] into the genome and insert in the middle of another gene and [this] could cause another disease. But we never found evidence that it would cause illness in human subjects.

The potential dangers associated with PERVs inform virtually all xeno research today. This has led to several intriguing innovations shaped by a new moral framing within the field. First, a relatively young vanguard of experts has spearheaded an internationally oriented ethics board that serves simultaneously as a clearinghouse for research publications and reports as well as a body that self-polices activities, steered by a strict set of ethical guidelines (Sykes et al. 2003). Second, substantial efforts to create PERV-free herds define a significant challenge in all five Anglophone countries where my investigation is based. Among the more unique responses involves the evolution of a moral economy of sorts, where various teams share off-spring from their swine herds with others around the globe, such that presumably competing labs collaborate on this research challenge.[42]

New Zealand has emerged as an especially intriguing site for innovative work by the firm I refer to here as Cellcraft because of the discovery of, and access to, feral pigs found on a small offshore island that are apparently descendants of animals left by sailors long ago who sought to provision the region with a ready food source.[43] In 2010 I visited Cellcraft, a small genetics lab that specializes in zoonoses detection, paired with xeno research. At the time, Cellcraft staff were determined to generate a reliable supply of PERV-free (or, at the very least, PERV-safe) porcine islet cells through a process known as "encapsulation," whereby insulin might be delivered to humans while preventing their immune systems from coming into direct contact with porcine cells. Cellcraft's founder, Peter Hansen, was a pediatrician who, in his words, "became disgusted with the effects of immunosuppressants on children."[44] In other words, Hansen hoped to circumvent altogether the need for allografting human organs in children, with efforts focused squarely on the possibility of injectable porcine cells providing a cure for diabetes that would circumvent both the need for a kidney-pancreas transplant and immunosuppression for a xenograft. Cellcraft researchers had already devoted over a decade of work identifying pathogens within their own specialized swine herds, partnering with the FDA in the United States and with swine vets from the United Kingdom to establish the strictest of evaluative strategies. By the time of my visit, they had already tested for over fifty separate endogenous swine pathogens. As their head virologist, Irina Milan, explained to me, "these animals are medical grade pigs . . . they are safe pigs."

Cellcraft's efforts are indicative of a new trend within xeno research, marked by the decision to work exclusively at the molecular level, where islet cell research is widely perceived throughout the field as the most promising area today. Another domain focuses on the viability of implanting porcine bone marrow in human patients. This shift in emphasis and scope is regarded within xeno as inherently moral on multiple fronts: it does not require the sacrifice of large numbers of animals, nor the extraction of whole organs from their bodies, nor, in some instances, even the employment of primates, because some researchers insist it is safe to move directly into human trials (and have done so without the sanction of their professional society). Finally, by working at the molecular level, the scientific perspective on xeno, so to speak, has been reduced quite literally to an invisible scale, such that the majority of activities occur not in swine facilities or labs filled with caged animals but by peering into the eyepieces of high-powered microscopes. In essence, then, the animal subject has altogether vanished from view.

The Promissory Pig

Today, pigs unquestionably define a prominent form of animal biocapital in xeno research (Franklin and Lock 2003; Shukin 2009; Sunder Rajan 2006). Although one still encounters baboons and macaques in xeno laboratories, they, like chimps, are no longer regarded as either financially or ethically viable donor species. Instead, they have shifted to an intermediate position, now serving as proxies for humans—becoming what Gísli Pálsson (2011) refers to as "border species"—in order to test the general responsiveness of primate bodies to porcine grafts. Meredith Kenyon, a Canadian and U.S.-trained immunologist who has worked in the field of xeno for the past thirty years, explained it to me thus:

MK: Many of us have problems using primates. They're *intelligent* animals. Their species, by choosing to use them, makes us uncomfortable. I certainly am. We don't eat monkeys, we do eat pigs. [Yet] our work is dependent on large animals [that is, primates]. That's something I still struggle with. [My work requires] a large animal facility . . . [because] baboons [are necessary] for xeno.

Kenyon's sentiments are most representative of those of North American and especially U.S.-based scientists, where regulatory apparati still permit the use of primates in research, albeit in more restrictive ways than was true forty years ago. Noteworthy here, too, is the focus on baboons (and not chimps) as human proxies. In fact, in late 2011, the U.S. National Institutes of Health ruled that it will desist in funding medical research involving chimpanzees (Gorman 2011c).[45]

As xeno researchers in favor of porcine grafts frequently tell me, "the pig is a purely utilitarian animal," occupying a rather unique position between food and pharmaceutical—or farm and pharma—production. Such experts regularly promote the promissory qualities of pigs by citing truncated histories of its domestication. As the much deeper archaeological record reveals, swine husbandry boasts an extraordinarily complex history,[46] yet most relevant to xeno research is the rapid pace at which science has shaped breeding and management practices over the course of the past century. During my visit to a California-based, university-run farm, for example, the director encouraged me to go back and watch *Old Yeller* (a film I had not viewed for over forty years) because the depiction of the seasonal capture and penning of feral hogs provided an accurate portrayal of husbandry practices of bygone days. The past half-century bears witness to intensified techniques designed to refine the physical and meat-bearing qualities of the animal, conducted, in turn, under the aegis of large-scale farming. As such, the contemporary pig is an altogether different creature when compared to its ancestors of a century (not to mention millennia) ago.[47] Today's pigs are overwhelmingly products of industrial production (Page 1997; B. Weiss 2012) that can generate hundreds of thousands of animals for consumption each year. As one swine husbandry specialist explained to me in 2009, "pigs are bred for their terminal traits . . . they're all destined for the food chain. . . . They are [exceptional animals when compared to ungulates:] they have the shortest gestation period, biggest litter, and [they are the] quickest to market of any farm animal."[48] The pig is a far cry indeed from endangered chimps captured in the wild, or from baboons derived from relatively small breeding colonies overseen by a hodge-podge of government, medical, and university suppliers. When xeno researchers speak of the promises of their efforts and the legitimacy of their work, the social history of the source animal itself inevitably shapes their moral vision.

All xeno teams that rely on pigs for research are, in effect, actively engaged in breeding programs designed to alter the molecular and physical structure of these animals. A longstanding practice that now extends back several decades has focused on "miniaturizing" the pig so that the organs of a full-grown hog are of a size appropriate for implantation in a primate (be it a baboon or, in the future, a human). All xeno scientists work painstakingly, too, to arrive at ways to generate herds that are free of PERVs and other endogenous pathogens. A range of additional efforts likewise target pigs at a molecular level, and among the most pronounced of these efforts focus on the basic mechanisms involved in antibody responses to tissues of foreign origin. One approach involves altering the genome of pigs such that they lack certain proteins that would inspire immunological havoc in humans (these are often referred to as "knock-out" pigs). Still others strive to make the pig more like us. As one graduate student engaged in xeno research put it, "These aren't just any pigs."[49] David Cooper and Robert Lanza (2000), two xeno experts, elaborate on this idea: xeno now has "pigs that look and sound like any other pigs. . . . But if we could look inside them, we would see something very strange indeed: *human* proteins on the surface of the cells that line the blood vessels throughout their entire body, in all of their organs. These are 'humanized' pigs" (43, italics in original; see also Sharp forthcoming).

During friendly bouts of intellectual sparring, those who favor pigs over primates may go so far as to claim that pigs are more appropriate matches for us than are monkeys or apes because the latter are evolutionarily *too close* to us. In these instances, it is as if their genetic, evolutionary, and social proximity threaten some sort of immunological incest (Sharp 2011a). In Kenyon's words, "There are many known infections [that can affect humans]; the closer the species the easier for them to jump from species to species." Still others go so far as to assert we are far more like pigs than monkeys.[50]

One such proponent from Australia is Peter Grimaldi. Known for his outspoken and somewhat renegade style, Grimaldi nevertheless inspires awe and admiration for his innovative experiments, paired with deep convictions regarding the need to keep one's finger on the pulse of public opinion as a means to insure ethical practices within the field. A nephrologist turned immunologist, he is also an inventor with several patents to his name. As he explained to me, xeno has reconfigured the pig's evolutionary proximity to us:

PG: I consider [the period extending from the 1990s] as the modern era of xenotransplantation. It's marked by a clear drive to the clinic, based on two factors: one, new and modern immunosuppressants; and, two, we can genetically modify pigs. [These together] will bring [xeno] to the clinic in an incredible way. . . .

LS: [Later in the interview:] But what if you make it a different animal altogether?

PG: [In] the animal experimental tree, [we move from] the mouse to the experimental pig to the primate. The fundamental thing about [xeno] isn't the experimental work, it's the clinical. There is no fundamental difference from other kinds of animal experimentation except the *genetic* modification. . . . What people don't understand is that the genetic modification is utterly trivial. We're made up of [hundreds] of genes, and [xeno involves] altering 1 or 2. The modification is quite trivial. [Now,] if you've changed the *character* of the animal—

LS: So, what about, for example, the spider goat?

PG: [Looks puzzled.]

LS: It's an animal that's been modified to produce tensile fibers, like spider webs, in its milk. Some people consider this disturbing.

PG: [Without hesitation:] You're [still] not changing the animal—just the milk. You're using its udders as a milk factory where the milk has special properties. It doesn't change [the goat]. We've [made use of] foot and mouth disease in genetic alteration and people get very upset about this because they have a poor understanding of what's happening. [As for their fears] it's all nonsense.

LS: I spoke with an animal activist recently who repeatedly used the language of Frankenstein to describe what's going on with xeno— she finds it very disturbing to take a pig part and put it in a baboon.

PG: Ahh, look, we eat 'em, we dress 'em up. It's basically nonsense. You can create a hysterical argument [very easily]. I [myself] could create a hysterical argument [without any trouble], and go print up a T-shirt and stand on a street corner and whip up some agitation. Some groups you have to deal with—it's all part of the terrain [of this research].

When parlayed scientifically, those who, like Grimaldi, advocate today for the superiority of the pig underscore its genetic malleability. In their shared opinion, pigs and humans have already been integrated in a way so seamless as to defy our ability to discern the transgenic animal from its original (or natural) predecessor. In the futuristic visions of these xeno experts, pigs might one day be custom bred to match the needs of individual human patients. An individual piglet could be generated in vitro to harbor aspects of one's own genetic makeup, the embryo then implanted in a medical grade sow, delivered by Caesarian section, and raised under pristine laboratory conditions until it had reached a size appropriate for its organs to be implanted within the body of the patient with whom it had been paired.

Imagining the Renatured Self

Cracks nevertheless emerge in the world of xeno research, as became clear during a plenary panel staged in 2009 at an international Xeno Society conference. Panelists had been invited to defend whichever category of transplant they believed should advance to human trials first. The opening question was most certainly hypothetical, given the range of immunological hurdles that continue to confront xeno. As a result, panelists essentially took turns providing updates on advancements in islet, kidney, lung, heart, and liver research. The presentations were followed by a rather bland question-

and-answer period, where society members spoke from the floor, asking for clarification on certain aspects of immunological work in ways that typified many of the conference sessions that week.

Near the end, however, a senior member with widespread surgical experience that extends back to the 1970s (and who had helped to organize the event) stood up and raised a more challenging question: "I'd like to know whom among you feels ready to accept a xenograft, based on your own research." The full panel responded with dead silence. After a long pause, the kidney specialist spoke up and answered diplomatically that many hurdles still remained before it would be possible to move to human trials; other panelists then followed his lead and made similar proclamations. Rather than sitting down, however, the senior scientist simply rephrased the question: "Yes, but I asked if you would accept [the very graft you work on]—after all, we have been hard at work in this field for a long time." It was now clear that he sought to chastise them for expressing reluctance, and someone sitting close to me mumbled something about the press being present in the front row. One by one, the panelists revised their positions, saying—at times in halting fashion—that, on further reflection, they each would accept a graft if it were their only hope at life, although one joked about the need for a hefty cocktail of all known immunosuppressants before he would do so, inspiring a smattering of muted chuckles throughout the audience. The questioner then sat down, seemingly satisfied. The panel chair (yet another surgeon widely regarded as a founder whose involvement in both allo- and xenotransplant research stretches back to the 1950s) closed the event by stating, "Let's try something like the Olympic Games—you can vote more than once." He then asked for a show of hands from the audience as he ran through the foci of the panel. The liver received zero votes, and only a few raised their hands in favor of lungs. The heart received three votes, the kidney seven, and a little less than half of the room voted for islet cells; the remainder, amounting to several hundred people, abstained. He then concluded, "Ok, so, we have the winner! Thank you for coming!"

These faltered (and rather obviously reluctant) responses to embody hybridity from within the very ranks of xeno science may be read in several ways. Clearly, none of the panelists felt that the necessary immunological hurdles had been overcome. I argue, though, that the panelists' unanimous ambivalence, paired with widespread audience reluctance, springs from deeper concerns about merging self and other. Ethicists have long engaged in debates over the social isolation and ostracism that xenografting could engender, alongside its potential to shatter the integrity of a patient's sense of self (see, most notably, Clark 1999; Vanderpool 1999). Just as the pig must be humanized, xeno surgery also requires that the human patient be porcinized. Although the latter term is certainly comical, it nevertheless serves to foreground the dead seriousness of xeno's transformative power. Yet as Mary Murray (2011) underscores, even islet cells pose threats, because their "diffuse nature . . . can appear particularly unpredictable and menacing"(112). In light of this, like whole organs, islet cells too might well be perceived "in emotional terms . . . as filling the body," albeit "in a different way" (112), "put[ting] us in danger of making animals of ourselves" and "the 'animal within'" (113, 114: see also Murray 2006, 2007). When taken together, the paired humanization of animals and dehumanization of patients are, quite literally, life-and-death matters. One need only consider the consequences of blood transfusion errors,[51] or the fact that organ recipients must take hefty, daily doses of immunosuppressants for their bodies to cope with *allo*grafts to realize the dangers xenografting bears. Hybridity as imagined by xeno researchers promotes the radical transfer of harvested parts across the species divide while inspiring unsettling thoughts about the transformative effects on the individual bodies of human and animal species.

THE TROUBLESOME NATURE OF HUMAN/ANIMAL PROXIMITY

Hybridity necessitates radical body breachings enabled through the remaking and blending of disparate species; when encountered within xeno itself, hybridity necessitates deliberate experimental acts designed to renaturalize source or donor animals so as to generate ideal matches for humans. Each species undergoes its own set of transformations under the aegis of this scientific discipline. Primates, like a host of other laboratory creatures, are highly valued as human proxies, initially as potential organ donors and, subsequently, as intermediate subjects in anticipation of placing porcine organs in ailing patients. Pigs are now humanized so that our bodies can respond to their parts as self rather than an immunologically dangerous other. These newly imagined, radical forms of embodiment insist on the blurring of boundaries that would otherwise distinguish human from animal. Yet such boundary crossings also raise moral confusion, a consequence most evident when competing social and scientific values assigned to non-human creatures collide.

Interspeciality—understood here as encompassing a breadth of experiences, ranging from human/animal companionship to the surgical or genetic melding of species (Livingston and Puar 2011)—is simultaneously intriguing and dangerous work precisely because it challenges the firmness of boundaries between animal and human, other and self. Animals are most certainly capable of becoming beloved companions, yet we nevertheless foster dependent relationships such that they must rely on us for food, shelter, kindness, and other forms of care. When humans and animals merge, such circumstances are read as unnatural and potentially monstrous pairings. Although we might care for and live with animals, what Haraway (2003) playfully references as "coupling" with "companion species" is considered at the very least provocatively renegade and, more frequently, pathological (or even criminal). The imagined breaching of the human/animal divide defines a state of intense desire within a science determined to fully naturalize interspeciality, and, as such, it rests alongside a host of other disciplines, including plant science, virology, and genetics, all of which strive in various quarters to incorporate materials of diverse origins within single entities. From the stance of xeno experts, even the most radical boundary crossings—as embodied in the spider goat or xeno's own chimeras—are celebrated as markers of exceptional scientific ingenuity.

If, as xeno demonstrates, the natural propensity in science is to remake, renaturalize, and retool animals for laboratory use, then such actions inevitably allow for some level of social intimacy, as evidenced by scientists' emotional and financial investment in specific kinds of laboratory animals. The procedures, regulatory apparati, and overall ethos of science mandate social distancing by way of an established evolutionary hierarchy (as with apes and monkeys) and utility paired with expendability (as with pigs). Such an ethos is not heartless (though activists I have interviewed would certainly regard it as such) as much as it is necessary for maintaining scientific rigor and integrity in the lab. Xeno scientists can most certainly celebrate the wonders of chimeras, though these same creatures (and associated imaginings) are regarded as monstrous creatures in other quarters, instilling "fears that we may be in danger of making monsters of ourselves" (Murray 2011, 109). Instead, it is the very nature of chimeras in xeno science that enables involved researchers to celebrate the wonders of futuristic, interspecies hybridity.

As I have sought to demonstrate, xeno is rife with moral challenges. Among the more pronounced issues today are those that spring from the dangers associated with zoonotic infections. Whereas the threat of PERVs drove activists to demand that xeno end, within the everyday world of laboratory research xeno experts approach zoonoses instead as defining a new set of challenges they must overcome in their persistent drive to rescue dying patients. And although in bygone days some scientists at least were driven by dreams of profit (as exemplified by XenoLife's trajectory), the majority of researchers I encounter today are so deeply passionate about their research that they readily share data—and their swineherds' progeny—in efforts to speed the delivery of their accomplishments from bench to clinic within a climate of scarce resources. Still others have shifted their focus from the whole hog, so to speak, to the molecular level. These scientists are often more broadly connected to others beyond xeno as a result, because their work on immunological tolerance translates fairly easily to genetics and clinical practice. Their shift to the invisible realm speaks, too, to a broader public captivated by desires to cure neatly, by injection, such chronic diseases as diabetes, lupus, Parkinson's, Alzheimer's, and cancer.

Set within an immunological framework, xeno experimentation involves altering, transforming, or tampering with the limits of that which is not human, not social, not self, not I. As a result, simian and swine species are each imagined as bearing an affinity to or some rarified form of kinship with us (Sharp 2011a). This preoccupation is of both clinical and social relevance. At the social end of the spectrum lie intense anxieties about the legitimacy of merging disparate species and, though muted in at least everyday discourse, these anxieties can be understood as part and parcel of the troublesome rubric of (re)naturalization, where no animal species should ever be fully changed, fully altered, or, at present, fully integrated into the human form. In this sense, animal activists—though understood widely within xeno as antagonistic extremists—nevertheless provide provocative insights that sometimes have served to foreground less articulate lay concerns and, in effect, redirect the moral compass within xeno research. Whereas activists declare how xeno dehumanizes us, xeno experts generally defend their transformative efforts as quintessentially human pursuits that could save patients' lives and stave off extreme forms of suffering. As xeno experts' more private sentiments reveal, however, it is one thing to experiment with transpeciality but quite another personally to embody the monkey or, for that matter, the pig. In the end, xeno science is about both the possibilities and the improbabilities of human/animal relatedness, generating, even among its strongest proponents, anxieties about interspecies proximity, the moral limits of transgenic science, and the frailty of the human/animal divide.

CHAPTER THREE

Artificial Life

Perfecting the Mechanical Heart

> The "bricoleur" is adept at performing a large number of diverse tasks;
> but, unlike the engineer . . . the rules of his game are always to make do
> with "whatever is at hand" . . . to renew or enrich the stock or to maintain
> it with the remains of previous constructions or deconstructions.
>
> Claude Lévi-Strauss (1966, 17)

Bioengineers are passionate genealogists. One need only attend plenary sessions at professional conferences, consult historical accounts, initiate web-based searches on such topics as "artificial organs" and "the mechanical heart," or access the archives of Project Bionics[1] to encounter a plethora of materials authored by specialists who trace their field's chronological progression by pairing inventors with their inventions. Bioengineering has long been dominated by men[2] drawn from a range of disciplines—including medicine, veterinary science, and numerous subspecialties of engineering itself.[3] Although many members are determined to stake claims by patenting their work,[4] they nevertheless describe their ideas and designs as evolving from the collaborative efforts of mentors who guide gifted teams of handpicked colleagues and students. Amid the swirl of molded plastics, translucent tubing, drivelines, pumps, and compressors, founding inventors' names are merged with those of machines: the Kolff Brigham Artificial Kidney and the Kolff-Akutsu Heart, the Liotta-DeBakey LVAD, the Jarvik-7 TAH and the J♥rvik Heart® 2000 System. Such mnemonics have given way more recently to corporate branding in a field now marked by such impersonalized designations as the Abiocor® Implantable Replacement Heart, HeartMate II® LVAD, Novacor® LVAS,[5] and the Freedom® Portable Driver of the SynCardia

Total Artificial Heart. A quick visit to associated university and industry websites reveals that genealogical histories likewise serve to foreground corporate ties to founding ancestors.

The emphasis on strides made by individuals—offering evidence of singular heroics—is widespread in science. As Mary Terrall (1998) asserts, this trend originates with the Enlightenment (and corresponding Scientific Revolution), when close associations were drawn between inspired men and the technical instruments they invented or employed. Terrall, a self-proclaimed science biographer, asks why historians like herself persist in focusing on individuals, "given that our discipline has moved away from treating science as a sequential accumulation of accomplishments and attributions of priority, associated with individual names" (2). In partial answer, she concedes that personal lives vividly illustrate the trajectories of disciplines; in turn, I would add that biographies, when (re)told by scientists themselves, uncover moral concerns, too. And, as we shall see, bioengineers are devoted storytellers.

As I illustrate in the first part of this chapter, bioengineers cling to this presumably archaic model of "sequential accumulation" when recounting their shared history. Following Terrall, I thus pose a related question: what moral tales are foregrounded when scientists' own narratives feature the accomplishments of particular foundational ancestors? Or, put another way, what moral issues are at stake in recounting breakthroughs within a particular field of science? Which deeds are featured, and which obscured? In my effort to explore these questions, I begin with brief accounts of two foundational bioengineering ancestors, Alexis Carrel and Willem J. Kolff. Xeno scientists also claim Carrel as a founder of their field, yet his animal experiments in the 1910s, by contemporary standards, verged on the bizarre (involving decapitated cats and the like);[6] his accomplishments in that field are thus overshadowed by those of other scientists who emerged later in the mid-twentieth century amid a flurry of accomplishments in allografting. In contrast, within bioengineering, the partnership formed in the 1930s between Carrel and the inventive aviator Charles Lindbergh was a hallmark of tinkerer ingenuity (see Bock and Goode 2007; Mol et al. 2010). Kolff, who was Carrel's junior by nearly thirty years, is widely proclaimed as the undisputed "Father of Artificial Organs," a phrase employed frequently at professional conferences, in journalists' accounts, and within biographies and obituaries of this formidable man.

Biographies, genealogies, and histories together provide an intriguing entrée into the world of bioengineering as well as a thought-provoking counter-balance to those encountered within xeno science. As I am often told by bioengineers, "I'm not a people person," a phrase employed to underscore their discomfort during social gatherings and clinical contexts where they might encounter sentient patients. They are, nevertheless, intrigued by—even obsessed with—tracking professional links within the discipline, whether through pedigrees of training, the histories of devices themselves, or, as I demonstrate below, prized experimental animals. As they trace these histories, profession-bound values emerge.

Consider the contrasts offered by xeno science. As described in the previous chapter, xeno professionals' narratives involve two historicized moves: the first collapses twentieth-century accomplishments with a mythological past inhabited by a host of monsters, thus demonstrating that ongoing efforts to create transspecies hybrids are typically human; the second enmeshes advancements in xeno science with others more widely celebrated within transplantation, underscoring xeno's significant contributions to technocratic biomedicine. These paired strategies legitimate ongoing efforts at transspecies grafting as both a natural human preoccupation and a demonstration of medical prowess. Although xeno science most certainly has its "founding fathers," xeno experts are more likely also to celebrate men known for breakthroughs in allotransplantation. In this sense, xeno science and human organ transfer embellish each other.

Bioengineers tell very different sorts of tales. Their origin stories feature most prominently the accomplishments of men daring enough to tinker with human life, their work exemplified by a range of astonishing gadgetry. Key elements of this master narrative involve an obsessive drive to accomplish what others might consider impossible, a fascination with what mechanical things might do, and a willingness to persevere regardless of ongoing failure. Although creativity is part and parcel of the field, ideas emerge simultaneously in a range of quarters, such that several teams (throughout the country or the world) may be hard at work on the same ideas. As such, artificial organ design fits more readily beneath the aegis of "applied" (and marketable) rather than "pure" (or theoretical) engineering, where ideas, devices, experimental animals, and, eventually, patients, define lucrative categories of biocapital (Franklin and Lock 2003; Sunder Rajan 2006).

Within the histories themselves, one encounters a propensity to merge the stories of men with machines, or inventors with their inventions. This elision generates significant repercussions for activities elsewhere within a field intent, quite literally, on merging human flesh with "artificial" implant, or what bioengineers playfully contrast as "software" and "hardware." In my effort to offer evidence of the morality tales embedded in discipline-specific narratives, I begin with a pair of stories that I myself have reconstructed—or "cobbled together," as bioengineers might say—from a range of professional presentations I have attended as well as biographies and obituaries often authored by bioengineers about others from within their ranks. Especially intriguing is the merging of inventors' histories with prototypes of their own design. As Terrall (2006) asks, "What can an individual life story say about larger trends or broader issues? How is science integrated into a life?" (307). In my own effort to "expand . . . beyond the confines of the individual" (307), in the latter part of this chapter I employ ethnographic data to interrogate moral values embedded in these biographies, with special attention to those that bioengineers assign to "artificial" devices, animal research subjects, the natal human body, and categories of suffering in a domain nevertheless viewed by many of its members as one marked by ethical neutrality.

ENLIGHTENED HISTORIES

One June 13, 1938, the cover of *Time* magazine featured an artist's rendering of the aviator-inventor Charles Lindbergh, who, standing at 6'3", towers over the relaxed and composed Nobel Laureate Alexis Carrel.[7] Whereas Lindbergh wears a layman's dark suit and red tie, Carrel sports a white surgical cap, a pair of rimless glasses, and his signature black operating gown.[8] Carrel's left hand carefully braces a fragile, goose-necked, glass contraption, a product labored over by Lindbergh[9] within Carrel's lab. Carrel, originally from the region of Lyon, France, had been recruited to New York City two decades earlier from the University of Chicago by the newly established

Rockefeller Institute, the first American academic establishment dedicated solely to medical research (Dutkowski et al. 2008, 1999). By the time Lindbergh met him, Carrel was widely regarded as a "versatile scientist" and "genius" (Dutkowski et al. 2008, 1998): at age 39, he was the youngest recipient thus far to receive a Nobel Prize.[10]

The device placed before these two men was a perfusion pump, its purpose to provide a reliable flow of oxygen and blood to an excised organ or tissue, sustaining its contents within a sterile and nutrient-rich environment until it could be surgically reimplanted.[11] By 1938, the two men were close colleagues and friends, having worked together for the previous eight years on this remarkable invention.[12] Lindbergh had sought out Carrel originally in 1930, shortly after the birth of his son, Charles Jr. Charles Sr. was driven by a determination to design an apparatus that might assist his wife's older sister, Elizabeth Morrow, whose heart had been badly damaged by rheumatic fever; the project would later transform into a desire shared by the two men to extend human life in a range of capacities (or, as otherwise phrased in the caption to the *Time* cover, "They are looking for the fountain of age").[13] Lindbergh was captivated by a respiratory device employed and invented by the anesthesiologist Paluel Flagg, who attended baby Charlie's birth, and it offered Lindbergh inspiration for how he might respond to his sister-in-law's medical needs.

As biographer David Friedman (2007) explains, Lindbergh, "who knew a fair bit about valves in machines, was puzzled that a mere valve in the heart—the body's engine, as he saw it—could cause so much trouble in an otherwise vibrant woman in her mid-twenties" (3). Lindbergh had several ideas that reflected an engineer's approach: "[R]emove and replace the broken [heart] valve, as he would do in an airplane engine; replace the entire heart with a mechanical pump—an 'artificial heart,' he called it—just as Lindbergh would replace a failed airplane motor; or insert a temporary blood pump, remove the heart, fix it, then put it back" (3). At Flagg's urging, Lindbergh contacted Carrel, a world-famous "*experimental* surgeon" (6, italics in the original) who had been awarded the Nobel Prize in 1912 for techniques in vascular surgery that later paved the way not only for heart repair but for organ transplants as well (4). By the winter of 1930, Lindbergh had ready access to dedicated lab space—and, moreover—to Carrel himself. Over the course of the next eight years, Lindbergh worked on a range of medical devices, learning in large part by directly observing Carrel as he conducted experimental surgeries on a host of animals (32–37).

Less than two years later, the notorious events surrounding baby Charlie's kidnapping brought Lindbergh's lab work to a full stop. The two men later revived the project two weeks after the discovery in May 1932 of the murdered child's badly mutilated and decomposed corpse in a wooded area not far from the Lindberghs' New Jersey home. Carrel had encouraged Lindbergh to return to the lab, suggesting that the work might distract the grieving father in the wake of this horrific tragedy. Lindbergh did indeed set to work redesigning and refining the pump, its associated components, and the techniques necessary to perfuse successfully an entire organ (D. Friedman 2007, 28–29, 54–60).[14] Although bioengineers are not nearly as familiar with Lindbergh's contributions to their field as they are Carrel's, today this device is widely celebrated within this field as an important precursor to various "artificial" organs, including contemporary perfusion machines employed in the excorporeal preservation of kidneys bound for transplant, alongside heart-lung bypass during surgery. As in xeno science, Carrel is widely acknowledged as a founding father of bioengineering, his prestige only further enhanced by his ground-breaking contributions to yet other fields, including tissue culture (he was the first to grow human tissue ex-vivo), mouse genetics, and transplantation (D. Friedman 2007, 4, 9, 11).

Only a few years after Carrel and Lindbergh appeared together on the cover of *Time*, Willem Johan "Pim" Kolff, a Dutch physician based during World War II in Kampen, a small town in the Netherlands, developed an early prototype for a hemodialysis machine (see figure 4). Kolff's determination to craft this "artificial kidney"—a cumbersome device cobbled together with an odd assortment of objects—was inspired by the death of one of his earliest patients, a young man who suffered from untreatable kidney failure. The imaginative artistry of Kolff the tinkerer is vividly illustrated by nephrologist Eli Friedman, who is known among bioengineers as the inventor of the "Suitcase Kidney," a portable dialyzer (see the January 5, 1975, issue of *Time*). Friedman (2009) described Kolff's invention as "a horizontal rotating drum artificial kidney with a sewing machine motor . . . attached to a bicycle chain that turned a drum . . . on which circulating blood with

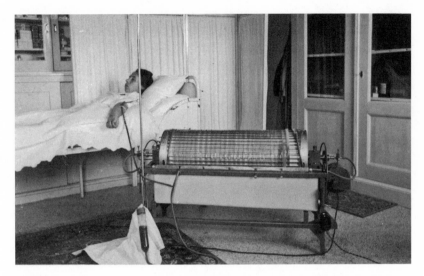

Figure 4. Nurse Maria ter Welle posing as a patient with the first dialyzer or "artificial kidney" designed by Willem Kolff in Kampen, the Netherlands, 1941/43. The device was cobbled together with parts that included a bicycle chain, a sewing machine motor, a water pump from a Ford Model T, sausage casings, a drum of wooden slats, and a tub secretly manufactured from metal salvaged from a downed German World War II airplane. (Reproduced with the permission of the Special Collections Department, J. Willard Marriott Library, University of Utah.)

cellophane tubing was exposed to dialysate in a 100 liter porcelain tank . . . with the tubing mounted on a drum built of wooden slats" (180).[15] Those who knew Kolff personally often state gleefully—and to underscore his ingenuity—that the cellophane tubing was in fact sausage casing (see, for instance, Brown 2009), which was made, as Eli Friedman himself explains, by the American Visking Corporation of Chicago for the manufacture of hot dogs (180). In turn, the original pump was derived from a Ford Model T, and the large tub was manufactured from metal salvaged from a downed German airplane and made secretly at night at a local enamel factory where activities were officially restricted to the production of pots and pans intended exclusively for use by the German military (180). After sixteen failed attempts over more than two years' time, on September 11, 1945, Kolff managed to save the life of a sixty-seven-year-old woman known as "Patient Nr. 17" who then lived on for another seven years (Broers 2007, 106–9).

Stories of Kolff as the intrepid tinkerer *par excellence* circulate widely in bioengineering circles, and accounts of his creative spirit in a host of domains are inevitably intertwined with the theme of personal heroics. Accounts of his early years emphasize, for instance, how Kolff's groundbreaking work coincided with the Nazi occupation of his homeland. As often retold at professional bioengineering conferences, Kolff, as a young doctor and postgraduate student, resigned from his post at the University of Groningen because he refused to work under a department head who was a Nazi,[16] subsequently moving to the rural town of Kampen where he went to work as a poorly paid physician at the town's City Hospital. His humanitarian efforts at that time were unparalleled: he is credited with establishing the first blood bank in Europe, and, while working in Kampen, he was a member of the Dutch resistance. As a doctor, he would assign more critical diagnoses than necessary to Jewish and other endangered patients so that their arrests and deportations would, at the very least, be postponed if not canceled. Furthermore, at one point he and his wife concealed a young Jewish boy in their home, later moving him to a caretaker's house on the grounds of a sanatorium run by Kolff's father when local police grew suspicious.[17] A detail often omitted from public accounts, ironically, is that "Patient Nr. 17," the first to be saved by Kolff's "artificial kidney," was Sofia Schafstadt, a well-known Nazi sympathizer who, following German withdrawal from the Netherlands, was sentenced by tribunal to several years' imprisonment; her son and daughter were similarly sentenced. Kolff's insistence that he treat her regardless of her wartime sympathies offers testament to his ethics as a physician (Broers 2007, 104–9). As detailed in an obituary of Kolff (and from Kolff's own report in Robinson 1976), "People begged, 'Let her die,' . . . But no physician has the right to decide whether a patient is a good guy or not. He must treat every patient who has need of him" (Brown 2009).

In 1948, Kolff's dialyzer was modified while he was visiting Brigham and Women's Hospital in Boston, and it subsequently became known as the Kolff Brigham Artificial Kidney (E. Friedman 2009).[18] Kolff moved permanently to the United States in 1950 (where, within the next decade, he became a citizen), taking up residence initially at the Cleveland Clinic (1950–67). By 1957, working in partnership with Tetsuzo Akutsu, Kolff developed an early prototype of a total artificial heart (now known as the Kolff-Akutsu Heart) that they tested on experimental animals; one dog survived ninety minutes with the implant (see Broers 2007, 149). Kolff then spent the remainder of his career at the University of Utah (1967-97),[19] where he established the Division of Artificial Organs at the Medical School and, a year later, the Institute for Biomedical Engineering.[20] All three institutions (Brigham and Women's, the Cleveland Clinic, and Utah) are celebrated today as leading centers in transplant research.

Kolff's extensive biography maps in many ways the history of artificial organs because he is credited with major breakthroughs in artificial kidney, lung, and heart design. His tireless devotion as an innovator is exemplified, for instance, by subsequent (though failed) attempts to design both portable and disposable hemodialyzers. As Kolff once explained, "I realized that nothing was very popular here [in the United States] unless it was disposable. . . . First, I tried a beer can to make these things, but it was too small" (Brown 2009). In turn—and as had Carrel and Lindbergh before him—Kolff set to work on a device that would inform the configuration of the heart-lung bypass machine. Kolff is also credited with inventing the intra-aortic balloon pump, a mechanism he devised in the 1960s that was first introduced clinically in 1968 by cardiac surgeon Adrian Kantrowitz.[21] According to Kantrowitz (1990) himself, by 1990 over 70,000 balloon pump procedures were being performed annually. Today this device is still used widely and regularly by cardiac surgeons at work throughout the world.

Kolff's most significant work, however, involved the development of a range of mechanical cardiac devices from which emerged those known today as Total Artificial Hearts, or TAHs, and Ventricular Assist Devices, or VADs (see figure 5). Once established in Utah in 1967, Kolff trained a seemingly endless stream of impressive young male protégés, who, under Kolff's tutelage (and, some report, exacting mentoring style), were determined to overcome the ailing body's natural flaws by designing mechanical replacements. Few would challenge the assertion that a catalog of Kolff's former students reads like a Who's Who in artificial organ design; furthermore, those working in the field today unquestionably garner prestige if at some point they had worked within or even visited Kolff's labs. In several instances during interviews, engineers have

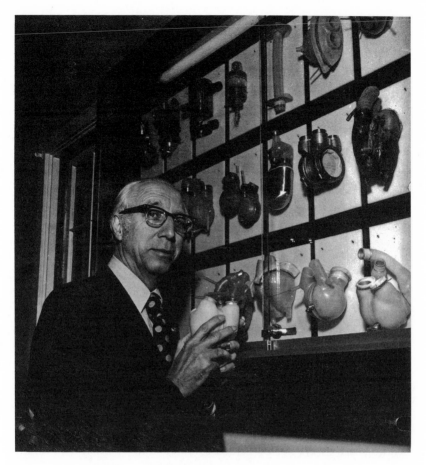

Figure 5. Willem Kolff posing in 1947 before an array of artificial heart devices at the Division of Artificial Organs and the Institute for Biomedical Engineering, University of Utah. (Reproduced with the permission of the Special Collections Department, J. Willard Marriott Library, University of Utah.)

informed me with pride that they can "trace a direct line" all the way back to Kolff; in one case, this involved a team laying claim to machinery currently in use in their own center that Kolff himself had built by hand decades before.

As evidence that Kolff was the purest of tinkerers, I am often told that he rarely claimed ownership of his work. He never patented his dialyzer, insisting that he preferred to assign the names of supervising students to devices on which they worked. Donald Olsen,[22] a veterinarian and long-term colleague of Kolff's, once described it thus: "We had the Donovan heart, the Green heart, the Kwan[-]Gett heart, the Jarvik heart. . . . But they all should have been called Kolff's heart" (as recounted in Brown 2009).[23] Among the most famous—though certainly not the only—artificial heart to be developed in Kolff's lab was the "Utah" TAH (sometimes referred to as the "Jarvik-7" after team manager Robert Jarvik) that was implanted in late 1982 in Barney Clark and in mid-1983 in William Schroeder, who survived 112 and 620 days, respectively, while permanently tethered to a driver system the size of a washing machine (see Sharp 2007).[24] Kolff was by no means the only—or earliest—person working on artificial heart design,[25] yet he is widely regarded by colleagues young and old as the "Father of Artificial Organs," a phrase employed regularly in tributes delivered at professional national and international conferences as well as in published accounts that appear in a range of transplant and bioengineering journals. Kolff died in 2009, just shy of his ninety-eighth birthday.

Of Machines and Men

Although I have encountered no evidence that "Pim" Kolff (1911–2009) ever met Alexis Carrel (1873–1944) or, for that matter, Charles Lindbergh, Sr. (1902–74), Kolff and Carrel bear much in common in terms of the morality tales they convey concerning "artificial" forms of body replacement. Scientifically informed transplant medicine, from its onset in the mid-twentieth century, has always been regarded as a heroic field, where risk-taking behaviors offer clear evidence of medical prowess and technological know-how, especially within the United States (Fox and Swazey 1978). Biographical accounts of Kolff and Carrel (and Lindbergh by association) are instructive in uncovering the sorts of details that inform the celebrity status of the heroic tinkerer. I identify three key commonalities here and then turn to the moral consequences of these narrative tropes as exemplified by my ethnographic data.

First, as European émigrés, both men contributed significantly to the advancement of American medicine, a well-worn story that is pervasive in the wider history of American science, for the twentieth century in particular. Each man held posts at what would emerge as important centers for American medical research, with Carrel firmly established at the Rockefeller

Institute and Kolff's own affiliations with Brigham and Women's Hospital in Boston, the Cleveland Clinic, and the University of Utah. All four of these prestigious institutions prized the men's abilities as inventors, and their associated activities eventually helped shape their technological preeminence—and that of the United States more generally—as world-class centers for transplant research and surgery.

Second, the conditions of war sparked the imaginations of both Carrel and Kolff. Carrel, as a French citizen living in the United States at the outbreak of World War I,[26] was called back to serve in the medical corps in France, where he established a hospital for treating soldiers with Rockefeller money. Working alongside British chemist Henry Drysdale Dakin, he developed the Carrel-Dakin solution (more widely known today as the Dakin Treatment), an effective chlorine-based wound disinfectant (Dutkowski et al. 2008, 1999) that saved myriad lives in an era that predated antibiotics. Kolff, in turn, pulled together a truly odd assortment of materials in his determination to dialyze dying patients; further, his devotion to saving all lives, regardless of political allegiance, underscores how he exemplified the ethical physician. The life of each man was also deeply intertwined with technological advancements that characterize the twentieth century: Carrel through a wide array of "firsts" in numerous fields and as a colleague and friend of Lindbergh, the latter recognized as a gifted tinkerer in his own right; and Kolff, whose professional trajectory coincided with transplant medicine's ascent (a field that likewise paralleled the Space Race in America).

Although each man was originally a physician by training (Kolff also earned a doctoral degree from the University of Groningen based on his artificial kidney work in Kampen [Broers 2007, 11]), both are recognized foremost among bioengineers, and in their own parlance, as "inventors," "tinkerers," and "mavericks" of science set on inventing "artificial" organs. The biographies of both Carrel and Kolff describe men who never seemed to *stop* inventing (Broers 2007; Malinin 1979, 1996). This propensity to invent new devices from a hodge-podge of parts is a recurring story encountered in the field. An internet search for "Artificial Heart," for instance, quickly uncovers the following description of the "toymaker" (Ohse 1993) William H. Sewell, Jr., as featured on the web page of the Eli Whitney Museum and Workshop of

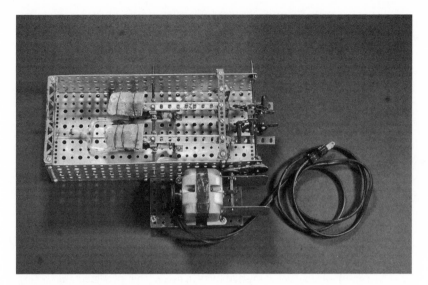

Figure 6. A component of an artificial heart designed by William H. Sewell, Jr., fabricated from a pneumatic pump, rubber tubing, a glass pumping chamber, a vacuum system, flaps from a toy noise maker, and, as shown here, an Erector Set™. This device was featured in a thesis presentation at the Yale University School of Medicine in 1950, employed experimentally by Sewell on dogs as a means to bypass the right side of the heart. For a detailed, first-hand account, see the posting "Sewell's Pump" by William W. L. Glenn, M.D., for the Eli Whitney Museum and Workshop, http://www.eliwhitney.org/museum /-gilbert-project/-man/a-c-gilbert-scientific-toymaker-essays-arts-and-sciences-october-3. (Photo courtesy of Mrs. William H. Sewell, the Division of Medicine and Science, National Museum of American History, Smithsonian Institution.)

Yale University; the original pump is now in the collection of the Smithsonian Museum (see figure 6):

> In 1949, a precursor to the modern artificial heart pump was built by doctors William Sewell and William Glenn of the Yale School of Medicine using an Erector Set, assorted odds and ends, and dime-store toys. The external pump successfully bypassed the heart of a dog for more than an hour.[27]

The flavor of this account underscores such qualities as audaciousness, cleverness, and imagination, or what Renée Fox and Judith Swazey identified several decades ago as the "courage to fail" specifically among transplant surgeons (Fox 1959; Fox and Swazey 1978, 1992, 2004). Such stories of medical heroics are very much a part of the lore of bioengineering.

The third key commonality is that the biographies of both Carrel and Kolff regularly emphasize how they bore witness to intense forms of suffering. For Carrel, this involved his surgical work during World War I and, later, as he bolstered his friend and colleague Lindbergh in the wake of his child's murder. For Kolff, it was both the routine of death in the clinic and the horrors of Nazism that fueled his efforts to fashion replacements for failed human organs. The master narrative that dominates tales told in bioengineering circles is that inventiveness is often driven by having to watch helplessly as patients die. Carrel, for instance, was driven to perfect forms of vascular suturing following the inability of surgeons to save the life of Sadi Carnot, the president of France, who died after being stabbed by an assassin in 1884 (D. Friedman 2007). Whereas this theme of the impotent witness certainly echoes the moral imperative that drives allotransplantation, bioengineers blame medical failure not so much on organ scarcity as on the lack of appropriate technologies and techniques. This then challenges them, as they themselves explain, to "think outside the box," "take risks," and attempt "maverick" solutions where they understand that "nothing is impossible," an amalgamation of traits that defines the core of the gifted bioengineer.[28] In turn, a bioengineer's work is never done, because every prototype or device can be altered, refined, perfected. Risk taking and "pushing the envelope" are frequently parodied in talks that celebrate the lives of foundational figures, who today might be pictured (through photo-manipulation techniques) astride a rodeo bull, jumping from a cliff, riding a roller coaster with an incomplete track, or leaping from an airplane without a parachute.

Biographies are, by their very nature, only partial histories, where the teller of tales must inevitably make certain (sometimes deliberate and strategic) decisions about which elements to include or exclude. My intent here is not to question the veracity of these tales; I am nevertheless interested in the erasure of certain story elements because of the moral understandings that then inform favorite tales of the tinkerer hero. Lindbergh—as one clinical researcher put it to me—"was a very odd man" or, perhaps better put, enigmatic: he was (alongside Henry Ford) awarded a medal issued by Hitler; he led an antiwar movement in the early years of World War II; he embraced eugenics; he advocated tolerance; he was accused of antisemitism. Other contradictions emerge from the lives of Carrel and Kolff, too. According to P. Dutkowski, O. de Rougemont, and P.-A. Clavien (2008), Carrel was a complicated fellow whose oddities—and politics (most notably as a supporter of Vichy France in

World War II)—have led to widespread neglect of his ideas and achievements in various quarters. As Dutkowski and colleagues explain, "The numerous of [sic] Carrel's contradictions remained too difficult for the public, and even many scientists, to understand" (2003), and he "appeared to be obsessed with 'the secret of life'" (1999), a long-standing interest that informed his work on organ transplantation. Like Lindbergh, Carrel exhibited a propensity for eugenics: his "dream was to conquer death. However, Carrel thought that immortality should only be accessible to carefully selected people" (1998; see also Carrel 1935). Carrel advocated provocative and, at times, disturbing ideas about the value of human life; in contrast, Kolff's early efforts at hemodialysis saved a Nazi sympathizer. My intention here is not to discredit the work of either man but to underscore that these are complex people with complicated histories. With this in mind, their biographies as recounted by bioengineers foreground certain values while obscuring others. What virtues matter here, and what do various erasures reveal not so much about these men themselves but of the field they so strongly exemplify?

THE BIOENGINEERED BODY

"I've never been a people person—I guess that's why I became an engineer." It is early 2008 and Kyle Arnold, a Euro-American man in his mid-forties, speaks to me within a corporate office cluttered with artificial heart devices. Having worked in the field for over a decade (and previously for another firm three times as old as his current employer, one that was renamed several times over), Arnold moves gracefully from descriptions and overviews of one model to the next, even though it is clear he is not accustomed to speaking to people outside his field about what his work entails. Without warning he suddenly ducks down and disappears beneath his desk, where I can hear him shoving about papers and boxes. He reemerges with two implantable heart pumps in his hands. "Here, hold this," and he places the largest one in my outstretched palms, putting the other—with a resounding clunk—on top of his desk. The device I hold is a thick disk of oxidized metal with two protruding hoses, and I estimate the disk's weathered casing to have a diameter of at least five or six inches. I am shocked by how large it is, and how much it weighs, trying to imagine something so cumbersome and heavy around my neck or, worse yet, embedded within my ribcage. The other device that now

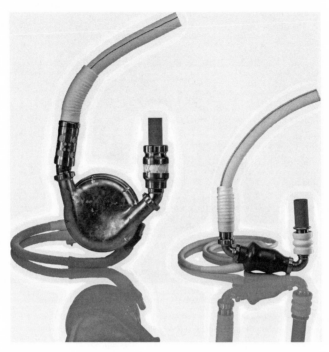

Figure 7. Examples of two generations of implantable ventricular assist devices (VADs): the larger, cylindrical Thoratec HeartMate® XVE, and the far more compact HeartMate® II. (Property of Thoratec Corporation, reprinted with permission.)

sits on his desk is similar in design, yet smaller, and composed primarily of sleek and shiny titanium. Pointing to the one I hold, he states, "that thing weighs a ton, and its external battery pack alone was two and a half pounds. This is how we started—fortunately the materials we have at our disposal now mean a much lighter implant, and we've shifted away completely from the TAH to ventricular pumps. It's still pretty large." This time he reaches behind him and opens a box sitting on his bookshelf, pulling out a palm-sized metal cylinder with plastic tubing emerging from each end. He plops this down in front of me, and I cannot help but think that I am looking at a piece of plumbing that might attach somehow under my sink (see figures 7, 8, and 9).

As I am frequently told by bioengineers, artificial organ design is a small and highly specialized world populated by a quirky assortment of "tinkerers" (Bock and Goode 2007). The youngest generation (consisting of students in

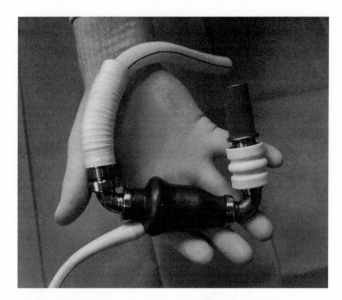

Figure 8. The Thoratec HeartMate® II ventricular assist system, displayed presumably in the gloved hand of a surgeon and set against a sterile field prior to surgical implantation. The image serves to illustrate the device's relatively compact size in relation to the human body. (Photo reprinted with permission from the University of Rochester Medical Center, Rochester, N.Y.)

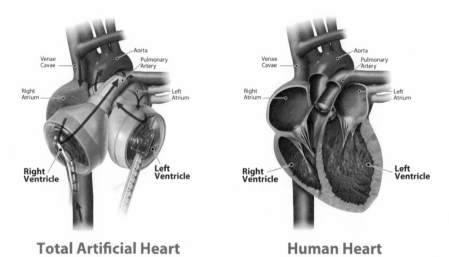

Total Artificial Heart **Human Heart**

Figure 9. Illustration of an implanted SynCardia Total Artificial Heart *(left)* alongside a cutaway of a natal heart *(right)*. (Reprinted with permission, courtesy of syncardia.com.)

their twenties and thirties) demonstrates radical demographic shifts in a field that now attracts women and an ever-broadening array of ethnicities and nationalities, many of whom choose the field from the start as their undergraduate major. It is, nevertheless, a field founded and still dominated by men who are now in their seventies or older,[29] the majority of whom are of Euro-American and European heritage, alongside a mere handful of others of East Asian origin and, even fewer, African-American or Latino. Bioengineering's founders started out half a century ago in a wide range of fields—most often medicine, sometimes veterinary science, and occasionally engineering itself—and they have unquestionably set the standards for what it means to "tinker" with the human form. Sandwiched between these two age groups is a transitional one, of which Kyle Arnold is exemplary, comprising primarily men who often began as classically trained engineers (with expertise in mechanical, electrical, hydraulic, and aerodynamic engineering) and only later drifted into what many refer to as the "bio" domain of the field, working perhaps initially (and in what most consider historically to be a transitional phase) within a medically oriented field where they learned about artificial organs.

Bioengineers of all ages are captivated by the possibilities of creating mechanical replacement parts for humans, and they engage in seemingly endless efforts to design, then test, reconfigure, then test, redesign, then test, and, they hope, market devices that can replace patients' failing organs. The process inevitably begins all over again, the engineer driven by an incessant and unsettling sense that every device warrants improvement. In this regard, each invention in artificial organ design in some way remains a prototype, an "exploratory technology" or "exemplary artifact that is at once intelligibly familiar to the actors involved, and recognizably new" (Suchman et al. 2002, 163). An inherent paradox in this line of work is a pronounced devotion to always changing, tinkering with, and perfecting the human/machine interface, paired with a rigid sensibility that the fleshy body should fit the mechanical prototype and not the other way around (Sharp 2011a).

Bioengineering—at least where artificial organs are concerned—is an eclectic field. Involved scientists' foundational training—especially if they are in their thirties or older—readily demonstrates a wide swath of disciplines: over the course of my research I have encountered thoracic and transplant surgeons, engineers, robotics experts, computer programmers, nanotechnologists, veterinarians, and even a philosophically minded nuclear physicist, yet the vast majority who embrace the title of "bioengineer" consider themselves first and foremost mechanical experts and, more important, inventors. It is not unusual to encounter individuals who hold multiple degrees or have at least some training in several disciplines.

Leo Navarro, when I first encountered him in 2008, was just shy of forty and already a rising star in the field. He explained to me that "years ago [when I was a postdoc in cell biology] I was having a bad grant day, and so I decided to 'reinvent' myself"—an apt metaphor, certainly, for someone whose self-designation is "inventor." Although he now teaches bioengineering at a prestigious university, when younger he took a brief detour and worked for a pharmaceutical firm, learning about heart valve design (an initial focus numerous interviewees reported as sparking their interest in mechanical organs and parts). Navarro is exemplary of a young and rising generation within the field: of mixed ethnic heritage; trilingual because his parents speak Spanish, Mandarin, and English; trained in medically relevant fields from the start; and married to a woman who is herself an engineer (her own professional trajectory marking a significant shift in a field that until recently was almost exclusively a male domain). Many others of Navarro's generation and younger have started, for instance, in a premedical track as undergraduates and then swerved into engineering when they realized they preferred mechanical parts to flesh, or, in the words of another female engineer of Navarro's age, "I always wanted to do research—I don't like having contact with people," a somewhat harsher version of a sentiment expressed by Arnold, above, who insists he is "not a people person." One also encounters physicians and veterinarians who, as surgeons, are natural innovators and so gravitate to bioengineering as a way to become involved in implant design.

As one seasoned engineering veteran in his sixties put it, artificial heart design is "the same idea in miniature" as one encounters in other realms of engineering. Artificial organ experts of various ages boast original training in such specialties as structural design, fluid mechanics, aviation, and electrical engineering, domains where I am often told one should "cut one's teeth" before getting involved in *bio*engineering. For instance, Arnold started in the aerospace industry designing airplane wings for large commercial aircraft, with a focus on air drag; he then went back to school to study fluid dynamics. As he explained, "I already had engineering training—I was ready to pick up the biology side." His "classical training" and experience inform his current work in bioengineering, a sequence he advocates is essential for successful work on artificial organs. In this sense, Charles Lindbergh is most certainly a kindred spirit, a man originally schooled in engineering who then turned to aviation and, later, designed a perfusion apparatus. In short, one typically approaches the body by way of mechanics.

In this light, an engineer might best be described as preoccupied with design possibilities and parameters, and such concerns inform conceptions of (and responses to) both human and animal anatomy. Whereas others working in the lab sciences (namely biology, chemistry, and physics) might challenge the idea that engineers are "true" scientists, engineers themselves regard the trial-and-error method of their field as both rigorous and flexible enough to stimulate the gifted inventor. Once, when I asked a structural engineer if he considered himself a scientist, he retorted with a snort, saying, "I'm an *engineer* . . . scientists take *forever* to solve a problem because they're so bogged down in the [experimental method]—they have to design it, test the hypothesis, etc., etc. Give an engineer a problem and he'll get to work trying to solve it through design."

This approach is exemplified in the work of Simon Fletcher, an upbeat, frenetic Euro-American who holds both M.D. and Ph.D. degrees. Just barely sixty, he has long run his own company while maintaining a part-time clinical practice and, as such, he exemplifies the tail end of a generation trained just after (and, for many, by) Kolff. Fletcher is a prolific inventor in several domains, having designed marketable devices now used in surgery, hemodialysis, and heart bypass. He also has first-hand experience in artificial kidney, lung, and heart valve design. He described his approach as follows:

SF: To be frustrated is a real *impetus*. Invention is really a science. You basically start out with a problem, you have a particular method, you think about the method.

LS: And do you hypothesize?

SF: The hypothesis *is* the method, for, say, that it will work or not. In a physical sense it takes six months. In an inventor's mind, though, it plays out in minutes. You keep going around in that loop, a couple hundred times. You think, then, ok, this is a good solution. Then you test it. You do a couple more loops, and then you get it right. It really is a scientific process.

From a lay perspective, presentations on artificial organ design seem to reflect little concern for human bodies: instead, they are eerily reminiscent of expert discussions in other quarters on how best to repair a sophisticated automobile engine, correct airplane turbulence, or perfect submarine propulsion—a sort of *Zen and the Art of the "Mechanized Self"* for the twenty-first century (after Pirsig 1974). One readily encounters this in David Friedman's (2007) description (cited earlier in this chapter) of Charles Lindbergh, who regarded the heart as "the body's engine" (3). During any professional gathering, discussions turn quickly to the dynamics of blood flow, rotor design, biodegradable products, and battery life. Among contemporary bioengineers, heart pumps are essentially sophisticated fluid propulsion devices, and much talk of their design concerns the ins and outs of miniaturization, velocity, structural integrity, cavitation, and corrosion, and the advantages of centrifugal over axial-flow devices, or pulsatile ("pulsating") versus continuous flow ("pulseless") pumps. Such words as "human" or "patient" rarely surface. Instead, the body is of greatest relevance at points of successful interface with engineered gadgetry.

As bioengineers always stress, "the heart is just a pump" (a phrase frequently employed by surgeons, too), and so replacing a natal organ necessitates designing a device that can move fluid—that is, blood—throughout the body's entire circulatory system. The artificial-heart-as-pump is a concept that relies on a very basic understanding of fluid mechanics: devices designed to move any liquid (be it water, sewage, oil, etc.) rely on rotors of various sorts (generally referenced as "propellers" or "impellers" in artificial organ circles) to control the speed at which the fluid flows throughout the system. Speed up the propeller, and the fluid moves more quickly; slow down or stop the propeller, and the fluid's flow slows or eventually ceases to move. In artificial heart design, one encounters a constant flow (so to speak) of discussions on how, and how fast, to move blood through the human body. In this regard, bioengineers are divided over whether blood should pulse through the body in a way that mimics the heart's activity (the "pulsatile" approach) or whether pulseless ("continuous flow") devices are just as effective—if not superior. As I describe below, these various designs have significant repercussions for patients who embody different kinds of machinery.

Fifteen years ago, artificial hearts were large and clunky like the one Arnold placed in my hands, and such devices could fit only into very large, barrel-chested men, ruling out opportunities to implant them in women and men of slight build, much less in children. Today, however, they come in a range of sizes and shapes, and advancements have occurred so rapidly that a critique I levied as recently as 2011, arguing that few could fit into the bodies of average-sized women, will soon seem outdated (Sharp 2011a). Nevertheless, the focus in the field remains the same, whereby bioengineering feats in artificial organ design are most keenly focused on two sorts of apparati: TAHs, which fully replace patients' natal hearts; and supplementary (sometimes called "augmentary") pumps that are implanted beneath patients' weakened ventricles to help move blood through their bodies with VADs (the most common of which target the "left" ventricle and so are known as LVADs).[30] Both of these apparati are employed in one of two ways: as "bridges to transplant," implanted only temporarily in order to sustain patients as they heal or await matching allografts; or as "destination therapy," meaning they are understood from the start as permanent implants, generally for those who have too many medical complications for them to qualify for allografts. One of the more celebrated (or, some might say, notorious) recent examples has involved former U.S. vice president Dick Cheney, who received an LVAD in 2010 as a bridge to heart transplant before receiving a donated human heart in 2012. Among the most striking characteristics of the increasingly popular continuous-flow pumps is that implanted patients essentially have no pulse (a characteristic of Cheney's implant that provided fodder for a spate of jokes questioning his humanity; see, for instance, James 2010). Patients implanted with pulsatile pumps, in contrast, frequently complain of the incessant noise associated with the external driver or the clacking of implanted valves, the latter generating a noise that can grow louder when patients open their mouths (see Wainwright and Wynne 2008; I will return to the implications of this near the end of this chapter). The latter example sparks the very sort of incessant tinkering I understand as inherent in the field: Arnold and others have invested significant time in correcting these design "flaws" so that the latest models, once implanted, can only be heard through a stethoscope.

Artificial Life

The ability to "think outside the box" defines the very essence of "tinkering" with the body's imperfections through artificial organ design (see Lieberman and Hall 2007). Within this realm of inventors, scientific ingenuity is firmly focused on the possibilities involved in making a better human by refashioning or bioengineering a natal body understood from the start as inherently flawed. The daily lives of engineers are replete with sleek propulsion devices fashioned from steel, titanium, high-grade plastics, elegant wiring systems, abdominal and skull-based output jacks, and portable battery packs strapped to the chest like gun cartridge holders, slung over the shoulder in what appears to be a camera bag, hoisted and carried in an ergonomically designed backpack, or dragged around on a trolley like a "wheelie" suitcase. This clutter of manufactured "hardware" stands in stark contrast to the messier aspects of human "software," or the flesh that makes up the natal body (see figures 10 and 11).

Involved bioengineers often speak of this "messiness" of the flesh as what drives them to perfect their mechanical devices. As I am told, the human body, as an integrated system, is prone to "failure" and "breakdowns," not unlike other worlds well known to engineers with its network of nerves (like electrical wiring), veins and arteries (blood circulation being reminiscent of plumbing), driven and supported by the heart, lungs, kidneys, liver, and pancreas (understood as sophisticated pumps, drivers, filters, and delivery systems). The fact that biomedicine already boasts an assortment of mechanical devices that provide what is often labeled "life support"—extending from the Lindbergh-Carrel perfusion apparatus and Kolff's early dialyzer to the iron lung and on to more contemporary machines, including hemodialyzers, respirators, heart-lung bypass, and kidney perfusion machines—lends credence to the shared sense among bioengineers that the mechanical enhancement of the human-body-in-crisis is a natural extension of scientific medicine. Whereas one is born with one's natal organs, mechanical implants have the advantage—at least from the point of

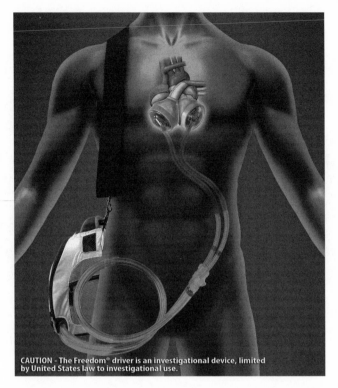

CAUTION - The Freedom® driver is an investigational device, limited by United States law to investigational use.

Figure 10. Idealized illustration of a SynCardia Total Artificial Heart implanted in a male patient, accompanied by its external Freedom® Portable Driver. Weighing 13.5 pounds or approximately 6 kilos, the power pack, which includes the external driver and rechargeable batteries, is designed to be carried by the patient in a custom backpack or shoulder bag. (Reprinted with permission, courtesy of syncardia.com.)

view of these specialized tinkerers—of having been tested repeatedly in laboratories and specialized assembly plants, locales where breakdowns can be repaired by swapping out worn or malfunctioning parts for new ones.

When asked what they imagine or hope for the future, bioengineers generally do not speak of patients at all but of generic humans as "software" "end users" in constant need of "hardware upgrades." They typically imagine an idealized world of "no peripherals" or, at the very least, of "trans-skin technology" where the external power source rests outside the body, relying on magnets to drive internalized systems, thus bearing no threat of infection because no implanted drivelines must exit, as they do now, through the

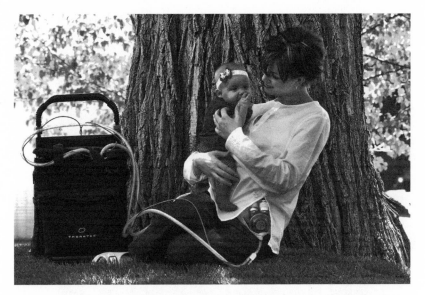

Figure 11. Promotional photo of woman (with baby known as "Bambi") displaying the portable Thoratec PVAD system, with a "paracorporeal" (meaning that it rests against the body) pump hanging beneath her shirt. To the patient's left is the PVAD's portable wheelie pack, which contains an external driver system powered by rechargeable batteries. (Property of Thoratec Corporation, reprinted with permission.)

chest, belly, or head. One engineer told me of his ideas for "skeletal-muscle power" as a means to drive a heart pump, and another joked about what currently would have to be a "very large solar panel" mounted on one's head. Unlike xeno researchers, bioengineers far more readily express a willingness—sometimes, even, with a twinkle in their eye—to accept these sorts of devices should their own bodies one day be in need of significant repair. As I have described elsewhere (Sharp 2011a), the work of the bioengineer is so keenly focused on the mechanical performance of swapped out parts that they speak of postmortem autopsies *of devices*, not of the implanted patients themselves. The bioengineer most certainly sings of a body electric.

In 2007, Fletcher invited me to visit his lab the next time I was in the area. His company is located equidistant between two Midwestern cities known nationwide for their state-of-the-art medical centers. As an entrepreneur in multiple fields, Fletcher enjoys talking about his work and, in a celebratory tone, whatever the latest advancements in the field might be. Upon my arrival, he took me straight into his lab, and I felt as though I were on tour with the Willy Wonka (Dahl 1964) of bioengineering as we circulated about a six-room, spacious, windowless complex staffed that day by three female technicians and several male and female undergraduate interns, the latter drawn from a local university. I expected to enter a space furnished with stools and lab benches, but in fact two separate rooms were each dedicated as electrical and machine shops. Fletcher showed me a plethora of materials related to kidney and liver function and surgical techniques, and each time we paused he would point out or hold up mechanical parts associated with an "artificial" organ, a phrasing he preferred over, say, labels that underscored their function (such as perfusion or dialysis). At one point he presented me with a small and altogether mysterious item no larger than a man's dress shirt button and said triumphantly, "a simple device that can make a world of difference!"

When asked how he became involved in artificial organ design, Fletcher put it thus:

SF: In college I was uncertain what I really wanted to do. I was on the fence between American history and theoretical physics. My talents were much better in physics and biochemistry. I knew that human interaction mattered to me, so I decided to be a doctor. . . . [M]y grandfather was a Depression Era doctor, so it skipped a generation—none of his [offspring wanted to be physicians after watching what he went through]. [But I found that] medicine was *not* theoretical but practical. In medicine, I liked gadgets. And I've [always had] hobbies rebuilding things like old cars, and I have a miniature railroad in my basement. . . . Most people who invent things really combine two things—theory and the practical. [We see] a need, and [we invent] a new technology. A problem in medicine is that it suffers from insufficient technology. A kind of "half-way" technology—if there is virtually no therapy [that is, no existing medical intervention], it may not inspire [others to invent]. It's the *halfway* that really drives you nuts. A lot of doctors have plenty of ideas [but they don't have the skills to make things].

I should note that Fletcher is hardly the first male inventor I have encountered in the course of this project who builds model trains in his basement, and the image of machinery assembled by hand speeding around complicated tracks that meander through miniature worlds in the intimate space of one's home (where one can be the *train engineer*) strikes me as an apt metaphor for the intellectual processes that drive these scientists' efforts. Fletcher's "half-way" principle is especially apt here: it is not merely a matter of designing something that does not yet exist; rather, it is the absence of something that should exist. This "nagging" feeling is something my father used to describe, an inventor in his own right who used to comb the pages of *Science* and *Scientific American* for references to missing gadgetry that he might design and thus help others advance experimental life one step farther.

Body Generics

When attention is focused primarily on gadgetry, however, certain moral shifts are bound to occur. Among the most pronounced in bioengineering involves the configuration of the body itself as a sort of prototype, and I have analyzed this elsewhere (Sharp 2011a). Very briefly, one encounters a moral aesthetic (Nicewonger 2011) that favors either *generic* (and thus *androgynous*) bodies or, more specifically, *male* bodies (most often healthy, athletic, and even, in some instances, militarized ones), either of which stands in for *all* bodies. The repercussions here are both clinically and morally significant. As noted above, until very recently most implantable devices could fit only into men with very large rib cages; anyone of slighter build—that is, smaller men and most women—would either have to live with chests that bulged from oversized devices or forgo implantation altogether. Yet another approach has been to connect devices (and VADs in particular) ex-corporeally, so that they essentially dangle outside the abdomen and, as one can easily imagine, render mobility next to impossible (see figure 12). As bioengineers often explain to me, the "math" itself can limit design parameters: that is, rendering a machine three-quarter size is no easy feat because everything has to change, including physical dimensions, flow rate, and impeller speed. And, oddly, when bioengineers started to move beyond the barrel-chested man, they focused their attention on pediatric devices, yet skipped over women's bodies. Very recently, a few firms have begun to design what some now call "three-quarter" devices; before, women had to make do with implants initially intended for children, remain hooked up to excorporeal apparati, or die.

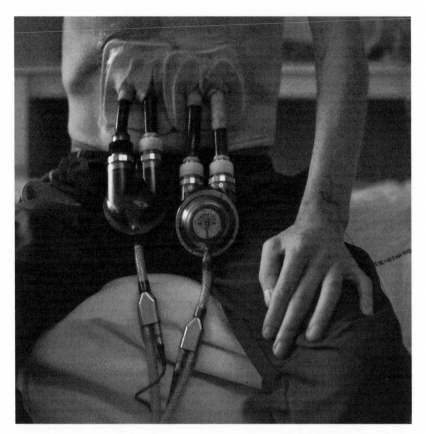

Figure 12. While awaiting a heart transplant, this patient was sustained by a double, external VAD support system that powered both his left and right ventricles. ("Ian's Chest," photo by Tim Wainwright. Reprinted with the artist's permission. Image from *Transplant*, a collaborative residency project involving Wainwright and sound artist John Wynne, through r&hArts at Harefield Hospital, Harefield, Uxbridge, UK, 2006-2007. See http://www.timwainwright.com/Transplant/6.html and www.thetransplantlog.com.)

When asked his opinion regarding the seeming neglect of smaller women's bodies in bioengineering, Barney Legstrom, a Euro-American structural engineer in his late fifties who works as a marketing agent for a firm that manufactures a remarkable array of adjustable and custom fit limb prostheses, said with a chuckle, "The engineer is *not* interested in solving every aspect of the problem—instead, if you can get it to work in most cases, that's good enough . . . [smiling] engineers aren't interested in 'the outliers.'"[31] To illustrate this, he offered a joke:

BL: A group of engineers and scientists are told that they need to cross the room; to get to the other side they are to step half the distance of the previous step.[32] The scientists start their journey, carefully measuring their steps halfway, then halfway, then halfway again and never making it to the end. The engineers take one look at the distance, take three giant steps across the room and say "It's a good enough approximation." When given a task to solve, if someone says "yes, but it doesn't fit x, y, z," the engineer says, "heh, I gave you what you asked for; if you want more than this then we'll go and design something else for that."

The gender gap within the field of mathematics, a range of sciences, and engineering is well documented, as I know firsthand as someone who teaches at a women's college (and as exemplified in what are known as STEM, or science, technology, engineering, and mathematics programs funded, for example, by the National Science Foundation). Fletcher is especially sensitive to this, and he actively promotes the efforts of women—in addition to junior colleagues more generally—through a range of innovative professional programs he has helped initiate. He explains that his awareness springs from the fact that his wife is a laboratory scientist and he has two daughters who are engineers. He offered this response when I asked about the gender imbalance in engineering:

SF: Gender—it's true, there are not as many women as we'd like. Maybe half of the biologists [that is, bioengineers] are female. And undergraduates—ten years ago this was not so, though. Nobody gets into artificial organs until they establish themselves [in other fields] as physicians or in bioengineering. We are starting to see [women]. It's funny, but women are more in [the] biological branch [of the field].

LS: Why do you think that is? Any ideas?

SF: I really think it has to do with toys. [He turns around and points to photos of his grandchildren on a nearby shelf]—look, my grandson is building something and my granddaughter has her stuffed animals. I think women enjoy beauty, and there is a certain kind of beauty that is in experimental science, and we're getting there. It used to be you would just throw things together. [But] it's a really elegant science. It's a *really* elegant science. A certain number of women have always enjoyed this.

Thanks in large part to Fletcher's efforts, the field's leading professional organization has begun to recognize these discrepancies and has made significant strides in recent years to draw young female scientists into the field, in addition to both men and women of diverse ethnic and national backgrounds. According to Leo Navarro, who teaches undergraduates, "Biomed is the hot topic. The [Baby] Boomers are going to die soon and they can pay for it. . . . They're going to want mechanical devices and the industries will bear that out." Nevertheless, female engineers, especially those who are in their forties or older, often describe the field as a lonely and even hostile environment where decisions to work specifically in "bio"engineering can be a "professional death sentence" if one has failed to "cut one's teeth" in the "classical fields" first. (The dangers of this choice seem to be dwindling among members of the youngest generation, who enter bioengineering from the start as undergraduates.) I discuss this briefly because the few women I encountered who were already established made direct connections between professional misogyny and the failure of their field to design implants that could fit into their own bodies.

Kay Blalock, who is among only a handful of women to have risen to prominence in artificial organ design, offered among the most articulate accounts of this. A Euro-American in her fifties, she reminds me of a rugged cowgirl and, as I learn in the interview, she did indeed grow up on a ranch, her mother a nurse, her father an engineer who specialized in irrigation systems. She looks as though she would be most comfortable in jeans and a tucked-in shirt with her sleeves rolled up, but, when I met her at a professional conference in 2008, she was dressed in sensible, low heels and a dark pants suit, a feminized version of the monotonous dark two-piece business attire 90 percent of male engineers wear to such events. In response to my question about the relevance of gender in engineering, she answered as follows:

KB: Engineering is all about getting along with the "Old Boys." As a woman they'll find a way to say to you, "You're not a real engineer, you don't know how to teach design . . . women are better at the 'soft skills.'"

LS: What are "soft skills"?

KB: That women are good at writing, articulating, negotiating, and working out problems, collaborating. But these are seen as secondary skills. It's all really about being able to make the prototype. In [traditional engineering] it's about fundamentals versus materials, applied design, making products. . . . You can't start in bioengineering and have street cred—"bio" is too "soft" to count as "true"—that is, classical—engineering. To do so is especially dangerous for women in the field. And it perpetuates itself—[I watch how] the Old Boys teach this arrogance to the Young Boys. Why are we doing this? Because we want to play with the Big Boys.[33] You used to see more nurses here. They're classified as second class citizens. Having them around breaks up the dark suits. . . . You know, my dad, who is an engineer, was surprised by my professional choice—he said I'd never shown any interest in taking things apart and putting them back together again.

LS: When I was in high school in rural Wisconsin in the 1970s, I signed up for Shop class, but on the first day the teacher threw me out, saying girls couldn't take Shop. When I asked why, he said I might outdo the boys and make them uncomfortable and said I was supposed to sign up for Home Ec.[34]

KB: Oh, but you would have threatened the boys, I can assure you.

LS: So, why did you do it—go into bioengineering?

KB: I wanted to help people. But aerospace, it doesn't go in the same direction as what I wanted to do. With that you help people in other ways of course.

LS: This might strike you as an odd question, but how do you think about the body?

KB: [Without hesitation:] [Unlike bioengineering] you're dealing with a more constrained system in aerospace [research]. The body is really complicated. It's a looser, more chaotic environment.

LS: Your current work is on heart devices. How do you think of these?

KB: Well, it's an organ assist device and not a form of replacement.

LS: And the heart itself?

KB: It's a pump.

LS: Ok, but what else?

KB: It's a very adaptive pump.

LS: "Adaptive," what do you mean by that? I'm not familiar with your use of the term.

KB: The structure—it's unlike anything else we have. You can't replicate it by replicating its structure. It's very interesting and unique—how nature decides to optimize something. It may not be the best design, it has its flaws, but it ended up this way. But you're making a mistake if you try to understand it through function alone. [I write in my notes: "I'm intrigued—it's as if I'm talking to an architect."] From a more holistic point of view, we could say it's the heart of emotions—as a scientist it's hard to avoid saying that emotions are in the brain . . . [but] I can't separate the philosophical from the pragmatic. As for religion, I don't really have much to say about this—I think about these things at different times and contexts.

Blalock's responses to my questions typify those of her (inevitably male) peers in the ways she understands and imagines the body, an entity that "may not be the best design, it has its flaws, but it ended up this way." Contrary to the majority of other bioengineers I have interviewed, Blalock's description did not end there with the model of the flawed, fleshy mass that defines what we are, because she recognizes its complexity and "chaotic" nature, too. Furthermore, she spoke of its mysteries (a highly unusual response from an engineer). She is thus a renegade in a double sense: determined to specialize in the "bio" domain of engineering while working among the more classically trained, and defying the assertion that her work is too "soft" on multiple fronts: as a woman and as someone who does not work in, say, aeronautics—and, thus, as someone of "soft" mind, body, and skill set. Blalock is cognizant of the body as enigma, and so she is a bit of an anomaly in the field in that she recognizes it is not merely about "structure" or form and function. For her, the body's management necessitates recognizing—yet also compartmentalizing—ideas that, in her own opinion, are the purview of philosophy or religion. In this sense, the human body drifts in and out of consciousness: sometimes it is there to be reckoned with because of the intriguing challenges it produces; at other times it fades from view as she focuses on the challenges of replicating what it can do.[35]

Even though Blalock initially entered the field because she wanted to help others, she was also among the few bioengineers I encountered who had any experience with what some in her field refer to as "implantees":

LS: Have you had any contact with patients?

KAY: I've met this one person with an LVAD, she was a young woman the same age as me, she had two little kids, a boy and a girl, and there were photos [of them all around her hospital room]. She died. Those kids—their mother died because the device didn't work. But most of my work is very simplified and detailed, so I have to confine [my efforts] to making it work, so that [the process inevitably] distinguishes it from the body. I can deviate even farther to a molecular situation of the body, to molecules—how much calcium [Note: I miss the technical details she provides here] and how does the device change this. So it becomes a very detailed analysis of the situation where you don't think about the body [at all]. [Still] it [the work] is always driven by this human need, but my problem is just solving the problem—to improve the devices so they last longer in people—it's a really broad, general goal. Because of grants alone we have to have a broad, a general approach [to our research problems]. When I started with LVADs, it took me off on a very different tangent, I had to learn how to design them. That was the goal.

Whereas Blalock clearly identifies with this now-deceased patient—who was her age and a mother (Blalock had a son age four at the time of the interview)—she quickly shifts back to an abstract notion of the body, a realm where she is most comfortable. In contrast, were she a transplant surgeon, she might have told me details about the patient's life and then most likely compared her case to others whose surgeries were successful and who had gone on to live productive lives. As Blalock's account reveals, the bioengineer is bound to principles and practices that call on or perhaps even require the erasure of the body. Although evidence of a patient's humanity—and of the suffering her death induces in others left behind—surfaces briefly here, Blalock nevertheless quickly (re)abstracts the body, reducing it once again to the parts that make up the whole by shrinking it down, in this instance, to a molecular level. As Blalock spoke of her experiences, I found myself envisioning a body that could appear and disappear as willed by the bioengineer. By no means do I claim these are immoral acts; they are, however, strong evidence of the workings of ordinary ethics.

Blalock nevertheless stands apart from the majority of her peers in that she periodically recognizes the body's—and the patient's—material and emotional presence. Whenever I attend bioengineering conferences, days can go by without my encountering any image of a human form except in the rooms reserved for trade show displays, where artists' renderings of generic patients' bodies give the distinct impression that heart replacement and enhancement technologies are embodied without complication, messiness, or pain (Sharp 2011a). In such contexts, the female body proves especially troublesome, as this discussion with Fletcher demonstrates:

LS: I am often struck by the absence of female bodies in images that illustrate how artificial organs are implanted in the body.

SF: I think it's modesty. You'd have to show her breasts. I just had a publication go to press that has an illustration in it. [He opens a file on his laptop and turns it around to show me.] It was a male, but a stylized one. [I write in my notebook that this color image is quite beautiful—on the left it shows a man from just above the groin up to the head, turned slightly, with an implant in place; the center of the image is a close-up, at the microscopic level, of what is happening within the bloodstream; to the right is the external drive system. I have written a note that visually "it is a spectacular image."] It's traditional enough in that it would seem a misuse of a female [body to show one]. Because they're really hooked up to a machine, and it's kinda crude [to do this]. It could seem pornographic. You wouldn't want to do this to a woman. If it's a male, you think, the guy had to choose this. There's a subservience involved—someone had to hook the person up, someone had to hook them up. You're more comfortable having someone who is *like you.*

LS: Do you mean that because it's a male you empathize with them?

SF: It's not a nice position to be in—it's kinda sad, really, that in order to stay alive you have to be hooked up to a machine.

Because the image had already appeared elsewhere, Fletcher's press hired its own artist to render a new version of the image. Fletcher showed me this one, too:

SF: Maybe this one is better—but they got the body wrong! Look, *the heart is on the wrong side of the body!* So we had to reject it, of course. But it's still male, like the other.

LS: Really? But, look, isn't there some sort of bulge on the chest that is reminiscent of breasts, and it has a sort of wasp-like waist, more typical of a female body with larger hips. Maybe this is what the artist was striving for—a more androgynous look.

SF: You think so? [He turns the laptop around to face him again and puzzles over it for fifteen seconds or so]. Really? I think it looks male. The other [original image], now that looks a bit more androgynous to me.

LS: But it has this big chest and the outline of the jaw looks male. I can't see any female qualities.

SF: Ok . . . but you can't see the groin, so doesn't that make it androgynous?

As I describe in detail elsewhere (Sharp 2011a), the bioengineered aesthetic is replete with images reminiscent of eunuchs—that is, nude male bodies, sometimes intensely muscular, that nevertheless have no genitals. Among my favorites involves a retouched image of a Roman sculpture that is clearly the torso of a virile young man sporting an external Berlin heart pump, his penis and testes clearly airbrushed away, leaving only a small, smooth, hump in their place. Yet, whereas the lay viewer would typically perceive this image as neutered in some way (and most likely, as Fletcher suggests, out of "modesty"), within bioengineering circles this sort of image is read as *androg-*

ynous. In other words, the default, prototypical, or generic form is a *male* body, and the female is, in Barney Legstrom's words, the "outlier." As a result, the female body is not only neglected but also fully erased from view and perhaps even consciousness (Sharp 2011a). This is not deliberate or premeditated but is nevertheless a potent moral act of exclusion that has significant repercussions not only for female engineers but for patients, too.

Animal Familiars

Whereas xeno science is intent on transforming the human by transferring organs from animals to dying patients, one might easily assume that animals matter little to bioengineers determined to perfect the human form by implanting a host of gadgetry. In fact, artificial organ research is intensely animal dependent.[36] Animals are, of course, employed in a wide range of scientific fields as research subjects (or, sometimes more appropriately, given their management, as "work objects" [Hogle 1995]). As I described in chapter 2, within xeno science primates and pigs are valued in a double sense: as potential "donor" or "source" animals, and as human proxies on whom to test the viability of xenografts. Bioengineering likewise employs animals, a practice that stretches back to the foundational experiments carried out by Carrel, whose labs housed cats, dogs, mice, ferrets, guinea pigs, and other animals (D. Friedman 2007). Certainly the presence of such animals signals efforts in science to spare humans from the rigor—and suffering—of device testing, but the notion of "proxy" connotes different meanings and sentiments here than those encountered in xeno science. On the face of it, animals in bioengineering are work objects that stand in for humans when procedures are life-threatening, and in this sense they might well be described as extensions of experimental machines. In the words of one researcher, "You want to be a good engineer and test [the device] as much as possible until eventually it could be put in a patient, and you need to do a due-diligence test with it in all prototypes." Yet contemporary bioengineers' engagement with lab-based animals reveals a level of sentimentality not encountered in xeno labs, where animals are kept at arm's length, so to speak, through anonymous coding and caging practices.

Whereas Carrel—and many others who followed him—exhibited a preference for domesticated household pets,[37] bioengineers most commonly employ farm animals and, preferably, ruminants, such as sheep, goats, and calves. Kolff himself appears to have initiated this practice. Herman Broers (2007), a meticulous biographer of Kolff's life, provides this dramatic account:

> [Following professional travels elsewhere in Europe and North America,] he begins his experiments on a cow. Kolff makes an appointment with the Food Rationing Service—it is 1947 and meat is still available only "on coupon"—to add an extra cow to rations allotted to Kampen. Whereas the town normally receives four cows for slaughter, at Kolff's request a fifth is now added. Kolff removes himself and his team to the abattoir where, under the supervision of the duty butcher, a cow is laid upon a platform one-and-a-half metres from the ground. Loudly lowing, the cow has been put under anesthetic but smells she is in an abattoir and is not prepared to co-operate with this unpleasant meddling with her body. In her terror the beast kicks and hits out at anything nearby. She shoots with a crash from the restraining belts and stands snorting and staring with huge, panic-stricken eyes at the recoiling Kolff and his confederates. This is more than enough for the butcher, who releases the animal from her suffering. A shot rings out and the cow sinks to the ground.
>
> After this episode, Kolff wisely decides to transfer his research to calves and dogs, and to proceed with tests no longer in the abattoir but in the garage of the hospital. . . . Here, in 1947 [working alongside other colleagues] . . . he has his first success with the heart-lung machine. A calf lives for a quarter of an hour on oxygen added to the blood by the apparatus whilst the lungs are out of action. The foundation has been laid for Kolff's second successful artificial organ. (121–22)

The foundation is laid, too, for ruminant involvement in bioengineering experiments under Kolff's direction. Once he was established in Salt Lake City, his preferred experimental animals included sheep and calves during experiments conducted most notably in partnership with Donald Olsen (see Broers 2007). Ruminants slowly became the staple of artificial organ research in the United States. The reasons for current preferences shown for calves and, though less frequently, sheep are sometimes serendipitous, sometimes sentimental, and sometimes pragmatic: a number of the leading (and earliest) departments in bioengineering are a stone's throw from farming communities, which provide a ready source of unwanted animals, and institutional expertise in large animal veterinary medicine only further facilitates the use of certain animals over others. Some ruminants can stand for long periods of time (and some will even sleep while standing), enabling easy access to implanted machinery. The docility of some animals matters, too. As Leo Navarro put it, "Calves are like big dogs. [Because an animal] post-op needs a lot of extra care . . . they become your pets." I have been told on two separate occasions by researchers that they prefer calves' temperaments to the "stupidity" of sheep, the " head-strong" quality of goats, and, though not a ruminant, the unwillingness of a pig to stand still.[38] Again, according to Navarro, "unlike other mammals, you know right away when a ruminant isn't feeling well because it stops eating and digesting," a tell-tale sign that can alert researchers, "calf sitters," and team veterinarians to how they can best manage an animal post-surgery. As he explained, "calves are really robust—they snap back immediately after surgery, and will stand up within only a couple of hours" after a device has been implanted. "A stressed animal gives bad data.[39] This is more from an animal husbandry model [than lab practice per se]."

Economics certainly plays a part in species preference. As noted in my earlier discussion of xeno science, farm animals are not as strictly regulated as those categorized as "lab" animals (for example, monkeys or rats), and so their care is, potentially, more affordable. I should note, however, that no one I have encountered in bioengineering has suggested this as a reason to rely on farm stock, although it does surface in xeno science. There is, nevertheless, a shared sense that ewes, rams, and calves involved in bioengineering experiments are already employed to serve human needs, and, at least where the milking of dairy cows is concerned, these animals are destined for a life where they will inevitably "interface" with machines twice each day. As I am often told, too, the animals used in bioengineering labs are deemed of little value by farmers and were destined for the slaughterhouse. As one researcher from a rural eastern state explained, "The animal [you use] often depends on where you are in the U.S. Here we [are all about] dairy cows. If you're a male dairy cow, you don't have much of a future! We liked to say that in some ways we're extending the lives of male dairy cows."

I am always stumbling across photos of male scientists posing with calves in bioengineering laboratories (see figure 13; see also Sharp 2007, 80).[40] The

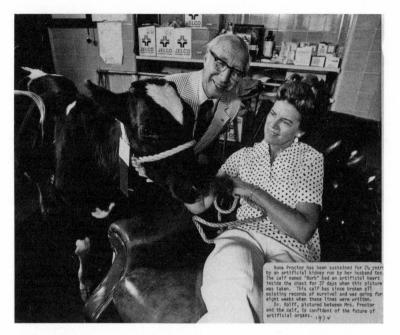

Roma Proctor has been sustained for 2½ years by an artificial kidney run by her husband Ken. The calf named "Burk" had an artificial heart inside the chest for 37 days when this picture was taken. This calf has since broken all existing records of survival and was going for eight weeks when these lines were written. Dr. Kolff, pictured between Mrs. Proctor and the calf, is confident of the future of artificial organs. 1974

Figure 13. Willem Kolff and Rona Proctor (an artificial kidney patient) posing in the University of Utah lab in 1974 with Burk the calf, a famous experimental animal subject in Kolff's lab who was implanted with an artificial heart device. (Reproduced with the permission of the Special Collections Department, J. Willard Marriott Library, University of Utah.)

propensity to do so stands in sharp contrast to xeno research, a domain populated with a wide range of creatures, including mice, hampsters, pigs of various sizes, and several kinds of monkeys. Although xeno scientists will sometimes pose with pigs (see figure 3 in the preceding chapter; see also Sharp 2002a), their public displays of affection for animals do not extend to monkeys, for instance. In contrast, within bioengineering a wide assortment of scientists have employed the camera to document their lab partnerships with calves, and many such images are now stored in archival collections. Among my favorites is one reproduced in Broer's (2007) biography of Kolff. It features Olsen in Kolff's Utah lab next to the widely celebrated experimental calf "Alfred Lord Tennyson." This doe-eyed Jersey stands on a metal platform and is housed within a narrow, metal stall held together with tape and rope; the roof of his enclosure supports a host of gadgetry and a large hand-written sign that reads "THE CHAMP" (figure 14). Olsen holds the Jarvik heart in his

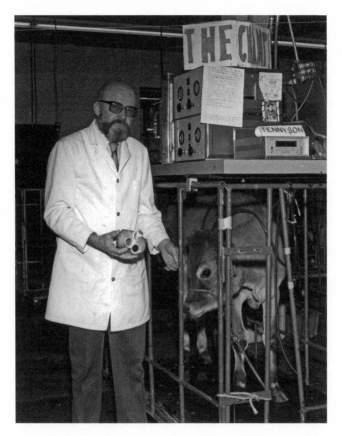

Figure 14. Veterinarian Donald Olsen holding a Jarvik artificial heart in his right hand while posing next to the widely celebrated experimental calf Alfred Lord Tennyson, also known as "The Champ." University of Utah, 1980. (Reproduced with the permission of the Special Collections Department, J. Willard Marriott Library, University of Utah.)

right hand while delicately touching the calf with his left, a pose that underscores the intimacy between the scientist, the device, and the laboratory animal.[41]

Even more intriguing is a propensity among bioengineers to track personal histories—paired with those of particular devices—through what might best be thought of as "calf genealogies." There are several famous calves, among whom "The Champ" Alfred Lord Tennyson is exemplary and who in essence served as a foundational bovine ancestor. Those most frequently memorialized—in addition to Lord Tennyson—include a calf named Tony who, in 1973, survived thirty days with an early Kolff device; several calves implanted specifically with Jarvik hearts in 1975, including Burk, the Holstein bull, who survived just over ninety-four days; another young bull named Abebe (after the Ethiopian marathon runner and twice Olympic gold medalist Abebe Bikila) who, in 1976, lived 184 days; and twin calves under Olsen's care in 1978, one of whom, named Charles, lived for seventy-five days with an artificial heart and then received the natal heart of his twin sister, Diana, who was sacrificed for this purpose. Charles was then turned out to stud as a dairy herd sire (contrary to lab protocols that stipulated animal subjects should be sacrificed within six months, once they outgrew the laboratory). Three years later, Charles had fathered 57 calves and weighed 1,875 pounds; with several daughters old enough to breed, he was then sent to slaughter. "The Champ" Alfred Lord Tennyson survived 268 days on a Jarvik-5 heart in 1981. Alfred's success story then paved the way for human trials, most notably the implantation of TAHs in Barney Clark and William Schoeder in 1982 and 1983, respectively. Broers (2007) devotes several pages to these calves as "hero[es] of the moment" (173), and a smattering of bovine biographies can be found elsewhere, including on a web page for the University of Utah, in a Wikipedia entry for "Artificial Hearts,"[42] and in oral presentations at professional conferences. During interviews, bioengineers often speak in sentimental terms about specific animals and about their work or encounters with these trendsetting calves who inhabited Kolff's labs.

These exceptional lab animals thus simultaneously embody three interwoven histories of calves, devices, and men. Nowhere is this more evident than in one of the more elaborate examples of animal-naming practices I have encountered, demonstrated by the following interchange with Navarro:

LS: Do you name your lab animals?

LN: Yes. You always name them. At Biotech University where I did my postdoctoral work, the Chief Resident has naming rights. The cardiothoracic surgeon—the Attending—puts in the pump. It's the Resident who opens and preps [the animal] and then closes. The rule was that you wait 24 hours before you name it.

LS: Why?

LN: Because things could go wrong and the animal could die.

LS: Are there naming rules?

LN: The best names have already been taken by other animals. You can't name it after someone currently in the lab or after a previous animal. There really aren't any [strict] rules. [Where I now work] we always name the animal after the previous [postdoctoral] Resident.

LS: So, in essence, students are conducting research on their absent predecessor?

LN: That's right [chuckles]. I hope one day they name one after me. . . . My favorite [calf] was Blimpy.

LS: Why was he named Blimpy?

LN: He was named after the sub shop across the street. It was open late and had great cheesesteaks.

LS: Cheesesteaks?

LN: Yeah, we'd always go there to get cheesesteaks, and so we named him Blimpy. . . . There are so many names.

LS: So, whenever you'd eat a cheesesteak sandwich you think back on Blimpy?

LN: [Again, chuckles] We treat them like pets. When my first calf died I was an emotional wreck. But it's especially hard on the calf sitter. . . .

LS: Who are the calf sitters?

LN: Students, 4-Hers from local high schools, lab technicians. You [have to] think of *Charlotte's Web*, but with artificial hearts—where you grow up with the animal only to see it die.

LS: Certainly if you have 4-H members, they're used to raising a calf only to then hand it over for slaughter. . . .

LN: It's true, if you're in 4-H you raise the cow [for exhibit at the fair] and then if you're lucky Safeway buys it, or the local steakhouse buys it. So then they'd avoid the steakhouse for a while. My [cousins raised calves when I was growing up]. You'd sit down for dinner [at their house] and eat a steak and someone might say, "Do you think this is Bob? Bob's quite tasty!"

The sentiments bioengineers assign to these animals mark a level of intimacy absent from xeno science. Whereas xeno scientists betray their discomfort when faced with the prospects of embodying animal grafts, bioengineers recognize calves and other animals as intimate partners in their efforts to design and test mechanical prototypes. Oddly, though, these sorts of sentiments do not surface as readily where human patients are concerned: once the device enters a human body, patients become "implantees" or "end users" who are there to test out the viability of the machine/flesh interface.

The Erasure of Human Suffering

A medical or scientific conference inevitably has an accompanying trade show, staged in a ballroom or suite of interconnected rooms replete with collapsible and transportable booths where manufacturers, hospitals, and pharmaceutical corporations demonstrate their wares, set against glossy displays and presented by friendly and well-dressed salespeople. Biotechnology conference shows are a tinkerer's paradise, where TAHs, VADs, and an assortment of peripherals rest idly on tables, inviting the passerby to pause, touch, and pick up all types of hardware; there is also an assortment of gizmos that hiss, whoosh, click, and beep, demonstrating how to perfuse a kidney or pump blood through a patient's circulatory system. Some even feature videos that loop repeatedly through surgical demonstrations of how to install various mechanisms within patients' bodies.

Whereas the bioengineer's marketplace is circumscribed by these corporate trade-show displays, just as often, and off to the side, one encounters its academic version, known as the poster session. Here, synopses of research projects are described on large-scale, glossy printouts approximately 3'x5' or larger, rendered on high-tech, large-format printers, machines considered indispensable to staff within any research lab. Photographs and colorful technical drawings punctuate text that outlines researchers' hypotheses, methods, and outcomes, and the authors—who are often, though not exclusively, rising Ph.D.s—stand at alert attention ready to answer questions posed by visitors about their work.

It is mid-2005, and I am browsing a poster session located along a side wall of a room dominated by trade-show displays. In the midst of these presentations is a bulletin board devoid of a glossy poster; instead, two rows of numbered sheets of notebook paper are mounted neatly on it at eye level and bear handwritten comments. A man who appears to be in his late sixties is seated before this display, dressed in a dark suit, a blue dress shirt, a navy blue tie, and comfortable walking shoes. He is surrounded by a cluster of young men in a semi-circle; their age and new yet ill-fitting suits lead me to presume they must be engineering graduate students. Several step forward to shake his hand energetically and to tell him how pleased they are to meet him. All are listening intently to what the seated man has to say. I approach the crowd and read the posted notes whose contents concern the post-hospital care of LVAD recipients. When I look more carefully at the seated man, I realize he has an implant of some sort behind one ear that bears an uncanny resemblance to a stereo jack outlet. Connected to this is a cable that runs down his neck and under his shirt, emerging again at waist level where it terminates in what appears to be a black nylon camera bag, the strap of which is slung over one shoulder and across his chest, so that the bag itself rests snugly at his side. I look again at the bulletin board and then back to the seated man. Only then do I realize that *he* is the poster session.

The following day our paths intersected, and I mustered the courage to request an interview; he gracefully consented, stating in jovial fashion that he was long accustomed to being treated as a "spectacle" and that he had an anthropologist in his family, so he understood the nature of my research approach. Soon thereafter, I encountered his picture in a host of places—in a video running within the trade show hall explaining the portability of a VAD device, in conference presentations on the superiority of continuous flow pumps, during a debate over how best to feed peripherals from outside and within the body, and in an ad where he is holding a hiking stick while standing alongside his wife within an alpine scene, offering a poignant demonstration of the promises a VAD bears in enhancing the quality of life of patients suffering from severe heart failure. The ad text read as follows:

Jarvik Heart and Pete Houghton Celebrate Five Fabulous Years
June 20, 2000 - June 20, 2005

NO DIAPHRAGM
NO VALVES
NO NOISE

NO SENSORS

NO SOFTWARE

NO CALIBRATION

NO AIR VENT

NO FILLING PORT

NO MAINTENANCE

NO MICROPROCESSOR

NO FLOWMETER

NO ERROR

NO INLET CANNULA

NO CAPSULE FORMATION

NO POCKET INFECTION

NO TETS

NO TELEMETRY

NO TROUBLE

IT

SIMPLY

WORKS[43]

The man described here is the U.K.-based patient Peter Houghton,[44] a psychotherapist, humanitarian, long-time health activist, father of several grown children (including those fostered and later adopted from a war-torn region of the world), and published author, including a book entitled *On Death and Not Dying* (Houghton 2001).[45] Much of our interview focused on Houghton's truly extraordinary and moving life history.[46] In 1995, Houghton had suffered a heart attack as a rare complication associated with the flu, and ensuing weakness led to his inability to work two years later. When I asked how this affected him, he explained that the worst part was the devastating effect of lost income at a time when he and his wife had two children at university; they were forced to sell their long-time family home and move into a much smaller dwelling. Near death, suffering from kidney failure and other serious ailments, a friend in palliative care said "you know you're going to die in a few weeks, but I'll see if I can get something for your gout." This same friend saw a notice at a local hospital for an LVAD clinical trial and asked if he was interested in finding out more about it. As Houghton explained, "I'd already worked in palliative care. I wasn't afraid of dying," and so soon afterward he ventured to the hospital to learn more about it. As someone who already had one kidney that had failed long ago, and the second now compromised as well, he did not qualify for a heart transplant under National Health Service guidelines. I asked him how he decided to proceed with involvement in the trial:

PH: I decided I wanted to do it [but it was] hard to get my mind around it. [One of my sons] said "do it, it's one last chance to do something for other people." . . . I was aware I was an experiment . . . I wasn't afraid. I was only afraid they'd leave me in a vegetative state.

LS: What was it like after the surgery?

PH: I felt like I was in a cocoon. [Living with the pump] was very, very difficult. Especially the first six months. I was so close to death already, but [I didn't have any idea] how difficult, how horribly painful [the recovery would be]. I had infections of my wounds, the cable came out—it was very painful, very hard. I was in hospital for [months, home again, then back again]. . . . I didn't think the operation had been worth it for three months. I had [terrible] wound pain. In six months I was thinking about the future. At [the one year anniversary] I walked 80 miles [over several days]. . . . I've got this extra life. I kept thinking about this Lazarus business . . . [after] I talked to my priest about it [who said] "Oh, you're one of the new Lazarus men."

LS: Do you think of yourself as "bionic"?

PH: [I'm] living as a specimen. [At first] I was put off by it. But then I decided to go with it. The media . . . won't leave me alone. I had to learn how to do it. I called a friend [who advised me] "lose your inhibitions and talk flat." It worked! When I first came to this meeting, I didn't expect [the attention]. I won't let anyone sponsor me [they wanted to pay my way here, but I said no]. . . . We [my wife and I] live cleanly. We laugh, and we love, as much as possible. It isn't always true, but we [try]. . . .

LS: What about survival day-to-day. What do you need to do?

PH: [I need] these [rechargeable] batteries—they're good for about [eight] hours, [they're] lithium batteries. And, no, [I] cannot plug myself into the wall. [But I also] don't need [some large bulky] machine to sleep. I had to learn that when I'm tired, I need to rest. With the pump you have windows. The pump assists the heart. . . . I am in slight heart failure all the time with punctuated rests . . . [At this point his cell phone rings; when he disconnects the call he turns to me and says:] That was my assistant calling. I must always travel with an attendant who makes sure I don't [take risks with] the batteries [running low].

A *Washington Post* reporter who interviewed Houghton two years later offers this even more detailed description of the pump: "[It's] a titanium turbine about the size of a C battery embedded in his dysfunctional left ventricle, the heart's main pumping chamber. It has only one moving part—the impeller that moves his blood. If you listen to him with a stethoscope, you don't hear the usual loud tha-thump-thump pulse. What you hear is a whir. 'Like a washing machine,' he says helpfully" (Garreau 2007).

When I met Houghton in 2005, he had already set a significant five-year survival record, and he worked closely both by the bedside and by helping to supervise an aftercare support group for other patients even though he himself struggled with depression. When he passed away in 2007, he was—and remains—the most celebrated ambulatory recipient of an implanted VAD device. As such, he figures prominently within a small genealogy of "foundation implantees," as one engineer phrased it. Widely celebrated by bioengineers, Houghton joins such revered patients as Clark and Schroeder (Altman 1983, 1986; Schroeder Family and Barnette 1987), each of whose hearts were fully replaced much earlier, in the 1980s, with a system powered by a driver that was, in fact, the same size as a washing machine.[47] The origins of Houghton's significantly smaller VAD device can be traced through a direct line extending back to activities in Kolff's Utah labs.

Implanting Hardware in Soft Tissue End Users
Bioengineers are, without question, experts on the inner workings of the human body; nevertheless, very few whom I have encountered have any experience with patients. As detailed above, human bodies are soft, messy, fleshy things that present design challenges for inventors whose moral responses to domains circumscribed by sickness and death involve ceaseless

tinkering as a means to relieve the pain and suffering of inevitably anonymous categories of "end users." In this regard, Kyle Arnold is an exception. Although he stressed (as noted above) that he is "not a people person," he cares deeply about patient quality of life, and his work in the past has combined design work with clinical involvement:

LS: Can you tell me about the early years? Did you have contact with patients?

KA: What were the patients like? They were extremely sick—they were usually intubated, sedated, with multiple drips, and in the ICU [intensive care unit]. They were awaiting transplants [but] they were not going to make it. Here's your LVAD protocol [that is, you had to work with the sickest of the sick, those destined to die]. It is a very big operation. . . .

LS: How long, for instance . . . roughly?

KA: It all depends on the circumstances—on the status of the patient's heart, what the illness is, how much damage there is; if there have been previous surgeries then it might take a lot of work to get to the heart. I'd say 4 hours, or sometimes it can take all day.

LS: Do you mean, say, 24 hours?

KA: No nothing like that, but you might be in the OR [operating room] for eight or nine hours—it can be really tricky. In a week they're walking and looking a lot better. Back then they would stay in the hospital [after the surgery]. They might be out there [in the hospital] for a year.

LS: . . . Did you ever have a chance to meet patients face-to-face?

KA: Rarely. I usually showed up after they'd been prepped for surgery.

LS: Meaning, you were there to look over the surgeon's shoulder?

KA: Yes, I guess you could say that. I was the one who knew how to install it. These were [clinical] trial [cases], and so the surgeon was learning how to do it in real time. They practiced, of course, with us there [with them] on animal models first . . . [and] I was always there for the surgical team in case there was a complication.

LS: Have you had a chance to meet patients?

KA: At first I was there a lot as the one who knew the most about [the devices]. I would see patients only when there were complications. There was one I will always remember, though, a mom with young children—everyone was really afraid she might die, and this was her best chance.

LS: And did she survive?

KA: She lived for a while, yes. I heard she improved and later had a transplant, but had complications. I don't know what happened after that. Patients are generally just grateful to be alive. But I haven't been to the hospital for several years now. I work here on R&D [research and development]. The hospital now has a full-time VAD coordinator on staff. He calls us when he has questions, and if necessary we send someone over.

LS: It sounds a bit like a service call.

KA: Yep. [Smiling] They're calling in the technician.

In the mid-1990s, when Arnold first started working in the field, awareness of artificial heart technologies evidenced esoteric knowledge shared by a small coterie of experts; by the late 2000s, I had encountered an increasing number of health professionals and patients familiar with VADs in particular as a means either to allow a damaged heart to rest and heal or to employ as a bridge to transplant in the near future. A dear friend of mine with an "implanted" or subcutaneous defibulator, for instance, now tracks the technology's progress at least as carefully as I do.

In some quarters, the use of heart technologies is driven by surgical desperation, as exemplified by cardiac transplant surgeon Stan Joseph. I visited his hospital inpatient clinic initially to meet the head of the VAD team, the circumspect Tom Riscoe. Within a few minutes, however, we were soon joined by Joseph, a man with an energetic personality and sardonic sense of humor who rapidly overshadowed Riscoe. Joseph's office was littered with knick-knacks indicative of his passion: hearts crafted from papier-maché, crystal, and stone, and a small sculpture of a surgeon at work on an anesthetized patient, the scene composed entirely of nuts and bolts. His walls had the characteristic photos of a surgeon at work, with this striking difference: Joseph's surgical blues and mask were splattered here and there with blood. I wrote in my fieldnotes, "There's yet another photo of a hand holding a bloody mass. But these photos aren't macabre but, rather, among the first photos I've ever seen that aren't 'doctored' with care, instead depicting the reality of cardiac surgery: it's a messy business. This Dr. is an unusual character." Riscoe, who was a new member of the team, stuck to what seemed to be a carefully crafted script reminiscent of corporate descriptions of heart technologies. In contrast, Joseph spoke off the cuff and in a far more cavalier fashion about the problems of supply and demand in transplant medicine.

As Joseph explained, he had been recruited two years earlier to establish a new transplant center in a medium-sized city in the northeastern United States. Although the city is known for its complex of teaching hospitals, Joseph soon discovered this was a "backwater locale that gets passed over for larger transplant centers, and I started to rethink what we were doing here. I had experience with VADs [at my previous job] but we only used a few, and temporarily. I've reached the conclusion that VADs define the future for patients like mine here. . . . We do a lot of VADing here . . . because I can't get donated hearts." Joseph is among the very few surgeons I have encountered in over two decades who will assert that "there will never be enough organs to go around," based on the stagnated ebb and flow of donated organs within his region. As he explained:

> SJ: All [of our patients] need their heart replaced . . . [but I soon realized] I [was getting] the substandard hearts. . . . I have to fly in to get what other [surgeons] have rejected . . . because of [my location, paired with] seatbelt laws [so fewer people sustain head injuries in car crashes] . . . and unemployment. . . . [Our center] suffers from the "flight of youth," meaning young people [who define the most desired organ donors] don't die in car crashes because they *leave early* in their search for employment elsewhere. So two years later here I am pushing hard to move from "bridge" to "destination" therapy. . . . We now have several dozen patients at home with VADs and we have no intention of transplanting hearts in them because we know now we can't get them. So I sit them down from

the start and I say, "If you want a transplant, don't come here. We probably can't help you. But if you're willing to take the chance on a [VAD] with the chance of a better quality of life, then we can help you with this." We work hard to be honest about what we can and cannot do. Acute patients [are put on VADs] temporarily until their hearts can hopefully heal. [But] the patients we're trying to target are chronic and can't get into [heart transplant programs]. They're non-salvageable. There's a point of no return. If we do an elective VAD, they're in the ICU for two weeks, they have an average length of stay in the hospital of two weeks, and then they go home. Long-term we're looking at six months to a year. They die. . . . But if I can give them an extra six months, they're grateful: maybe it's so they can see their first grandchild, or go to their kid's graduation.

LS: How do patients respond to living with a VAD?

SJ: Acute patients wake up and are shocked by what has happened—they may not have had a [cardiac episode ever in their lives] and then they wake up and learn they have this machine inside them. . . . I talk to the psychologists a lot about this. . . . The chronic patients have known about and lived with heart disease for a very long time, and they know they're in bad shape and are dying. But the technology can only do so much because they have all sorts of health problems that stem from an ailing heart. So, on the one hand, they can't necessarily ever get a transplant, and their bodies may be so ravaged by the byproducts of heart disease that they may not do well with a pump; on the other, when the pump is installed as an "elective VAD" they really get the idea, and they take it in stride, because they've been so sick before and if the VAD works they can't believe they're up and walking around again. . . . I talk about this a lot with other [surgeons]. I have a friend who says "I can keep a Class 4 heart patient [alive] for a year." I tell him, "Sure, but let me tie a bag around your head for a year" [i.e., because they will still have difficulty breathing, making every breath a form of torture]. . . . We have [dozens of] patients home right now. . . . In terms of quality of life, we win hands down.

LS: You mentioned you talk to psychologists about patients' experiences. Can you elaborate a bit on this?

SJ: I talk to the psychologists [because] I'm interested in the psychological [components of their experiences]. I want to know about the social standpoint of what it's like having a driveline coming out of them. What does a cardiologist think about it? To engineers, it's no big deal. But [we also know that] if you have an acute shock—it's as if they were struck by lightening [i.e, waking up and learning you have a VAD implant is a major shock]—it's something you never expected. With chronic, they can't even butter their toast. . . . I say to patients, I'm going to give you a choice—you can have lung cancer, pancreatic cancer, AIDS, or heart failure. People *overwhelmingly* choose heart failure. They don't know how bad it is! [But] it is a terminal disease! [He then pulls out two photos, the first looks like a pale, ageless, anorexic woman, yet I learn it is a man; the second is a rotund man in his sixties—no matter how hard I look I cannot perceive of these two as the same person.] I like to compare it to those photos—what do you see? . . . I say, "I'd like you to look at these photos because they say it all—they illustrate it better than anything else can. This is *not* an optical illusion."

[For patients,] it all has to do with the peripherals. I have a patient who calls me now and says his golf swing is off because the driveline is getting in the way. Imagine! Another has figured out how to swim—he gets in the water to swim laps and a friend walks along the side of the pool holding the controls. I have another patient who goes out—he goes out *alone*—on his 4-wheeler [ATV or all terrain vehicle]. What happens if he crashes and he's out there alone?

LS: I guess he'd die if his power runs out.

SJ: Yes—*he could die*, but this is the way he wants to be able to live his life now. You see, the family's reaction really varies [too]. Some feel imprisoned, some paralyzed by the device. It can be *hell* for a family member. The wife of one patient says "I have to be by his side 24/7" and it's killing *her.*

LS: How about patients—how do they think about the mechanism inside of them?

SJ: [It depends on the model. With one] they all complained about the *noise*. They hear it [all the time]. For some it becomes—they got used to it. After transplant, those patients say "I miss it." This really surprised me. With some devices, some people can hear a hum inside them. But for the acute [patient] it's really different. Bam! They've never had heart failure.

Joseph's sentiments are indeed a far cry from those expressed by many an engineer whose role, in Kyle Arnold's words, more closely approximates that of the "technician," a trouble shooter and repairman who provides expert, pragmatic knowledge on how to save a life. Joseph's detailed responses spring most certainly from his day-to-day clinical encounters with patients; he is nevertheless an outlier in terms of his ongoing efforts to understand the psychological effects of VAD implantation, or what sociologist James Hughes (2004)—who consulted closely with Houghton—describes as the life of the "citizen cyborg." As Houghton's own testimonies in a range of interview contexts underscore, daily trials associated with LVADs encompass not only physical pain, surgical complications, fear, and depression but also surreal experiences that included fighting off a mugger who mistook his power pack for a camera bag (and then possessing the necessary self-composure to plug himself back in before collapsing; see Garreau 2007). At one point, Houghton generated significant distress in an attending physician who found it incomprehensible that a man who had no pulse could nevertheless sit up on a bed in an emergency room and converse without difficulty.

Such an experience was recounted to me by Kelly Morsy, a young medical student doing her rotation in critical care in a teaching hospital in New York City:

KM: I have worked with a few [patients with VADs] in the ICU. One post-surgical patient was awake and alert [even though what] he had could have been a fatal rhythm. [But] he was awake and alert. . . . This is a classic case of a patient who should be dead but they're sitting up and eating a popsicle or talking to you because the

VAD works in ways very different from the natal heart. . . . [Some-
one from the] Telemetry [Department that monitors the devices]
showed up because they got an alarm. [The patient] had an axial
flow device and [Telemetry] called me in because . . . they are
required to call in a physician.

Whereas the relative silence of an axial flow (that is, "pulseless") pump
generates anxiety in the novice physician, some patients themselves speak
of the annoying and even maddening qualities associated with the clacking
of heart valves in some devices (a sound that, at least in earlier models, is
more audible to bystanders at those moments when patients open their
mouths). For others, it is the incessant floopity-floop-floop of an external
drive system. The team of sound artist John Wynne and photographer Tim
Wainwright assembled an extraordinary corpus of work throughout a year-
long artists' residency at Harefield Hospital in the United Kingdom, where
their interviews with patients revealed, for example, a woman's attempts to
cope with a pump's unremitting noise by transforming it in her mind into
more bearable bird calls, or a man's careful tracking of a pump's wheezing
rhythm whose repetitive, four-beat cycle offered him constant proof that
without it "I would be dead by now."[48]

THE FANTASY OF ETHICAL NEUTRALITY

Throughout the course of my research, I have often asked people what they
consider to be the most pressing ethical parameters of experimental organ
replacement. Interestingly, surveys, informal interviews, and conversations
with lay parties expose a widely shared sentiment that whereas the employment of animals in xeno research is fraught with ethical challenges—because
the animals themselves would suffer, as would patients forced to cope with
newly configured bodies that are no longer wholly human—mechanical
implants are somehow imagined as "ethics free," as one of my own students
once phrased it. To be more precise, as explained to me by an engineer I
encountered in 2009 who co-taught a graduate-level ethics course at a midwestern school, "Just because the FDA says it's o.k. doesn't mean it is o.k. to
try something. But nothing is risk free. Ethics—the ethics are not complicated. It's not the same as with xenotransplantation." The presumably inert

qualities we assign to plastic, titanium, surgical Velcro, electrical lines, jacks, stents, rotors, and drivers lead to a widespread bracketing out of the moral consequences that plague the life of the "citizen cyborg" (again, see Hughes 2004; see also Gray 2001). Within bioengineering itself, the genea-logical blending of inventors with their inventions, and the subsequent inte-gration of animal histories, facilitates widespread neglect of individual stories. Only the names of the most remarkable patients (Clark, Schroeder, Houghton) remain in the public record or, for that matter, are recalled with any regularity by engineers themselves. Others fall into obscurity. As exem-plified in the following vignette, what emerges is an erasure of human suffering.

It is mid-2009, and I am only partially listening to a conference session presentation on the "chronic in-vivo performance" of a particular LVAD device. The speaker is an American M.D./Ph.D. who is rattling on about bearing cones, sub-miniature permanent blood pumps, pin and sleeve junc-tures, and low friction results that characterize slow speed function as recorded by his surgical team and associated Midwestern hospital-based lab. The presentation is what bioengineers generally label as device "autopsies": pathology reports on the wear and tear of mechanical implants that have been "explanted" from various patients, or what Kay Blalock and others describe as "end users." This is one of many such autopsy overviews I have heard this week, and I wait somewhat impatiently for a later paper by Kelly Morsy. I am suddenly aware, however, that the speaker is describing find-ings associated with two pediatric devices, one of which had been "explanted" from a toddler, the other an infant, and I bolt to attention to learn if the children had survived and gone on either to receive allografts or perhaps had healed once "explanted" and gone home to join their respective families. It is impossible to tell. The speaker drones on: "There is no failure of the pump due to the bearings at all . . . although the little pump doesn't pump all that [an adult] pump would pump . . . it's all about what we wish to accomplish with these pumps." I find myself thinking about a book from my childhood, *The Little Engine That Could*. We're now looking at color graphs of flow output, and then a picture of pin bearings "removed from the longest implantee in years." A chill runs up my spine: he is speaking of Peter Houghton.

As an ethnographer, one inevitably encounters remarkable people whom one can never forget. Perhaps the ethnographer witnesses them accomplishing extraordinary feats, surviving terrible adversities, or even doing terrible things. These are people whose lives occasionally offer cautionary moral tales for us, too. Within my discipline, we sometimes label such remarkable people "key informants," although this phrase fails to capture how deeply they might touch—and transform—our own lives as a result. For me, Houghton was such a person. At the time of this presentation, I did not know that Houghton had passed away; after hearing the speaker's remark regarding "the longest implantee in years," I was overcome with a deep sadness. Soon growing impatient with the presentation, I fidgeted in my seat until the talk was over. During the brief break that followed, I approached the speaker and asked him if he was indeed referring to Houghton, and he answered in the affirmative. I explained I had met Houghton once; what followed was an even more involved, clinical account of the autopsy's findings from him, alongside a few details on the circumstances of Houghton's death, whose end-of-life treatment proved especially complicated because he was supposedly first admitted to a hospital where staff were unfamiliar with VADs.[49] The presenter hypothesized that, based on conversations with those familiar with "the case," such circumstances may well have contributed to Houghton's death; he then shifted back to the subject of how Houghton's device had weathered years of constant use. My stomach in knots, I returned to my seat and, sitting once again in a darkened conference room, I listened while in a state best described as half-hearted, struggling to stay focused enough to jot down notes on Morsy's advice on how to provide optimal clinical support to postoperative LVAD recipients.

Attention to the ethics of device design, as part and parcel of the ethics of care, is nevertheless slowly making headway in university curricula. Within my own university (where I sometimes serve as a guest speaker within the engineering program), discussions inevitably boil down to "should we do it or not?" As Leo Navarro informed me at one point, "Ethics is part of the accreditation process for engineering. [When] testing [devices] we have to go into people. Ethics is usually part of a design class curriculum. In my engineering class, my students have to imagine they are working for industry, and they have to write two letters: one is the recall letter to a hospital, the other is the recall letter to a patient." At the time at which I write this chapter, however, Navarro remains an "outlier." As I describe elsewhere (Sharp 2009), an ability to conceive of patient suffering may be blocked at every turn by the narrow parameters of the moral imagination in transplant engineering, where the word "suffering" itself is denied or, even, taboo. When patients are "soft tissue" "end users" with "dysfunctional" hearts whose own "explanted" devices warrant careful "autopsy" reports, such framing leaves little room for the acknowledgment of a patient's physical pain, depression, or existential angst associated with a newly configured, bionic existence. Instead, the moral imaginative qualities of bioengineering are driven by celebrations of scientific ingenuity and prowess, understood as a willingness to tinker endlessly with the human form and thus to work, and think, "outside the box." Such efforts to make a better human serve to naturalize widespread neglect of both profound and peculiar causes of human suffering.

CHAPTER FOUR

Temporality and Social Desire in Anticipatory Science

Chancy origins . . . match chancy futures.

Marilyn Strathern (1992, 177)

Experimental science is by definition an *anticipatory* enterprise. Whereas funding proposals and associated research design are framed and driven by clearly articulated goals, outcomes are always hypothetical and, thus, unknown. In short, the black box of science obscures future knowledge, making way for imagination and desire. A host of technical questions dog those scientists engaged in experimental transplant research who are intent on redirecting clinical practices. For instance, how close, truly, is the pig's genome to that of *Homo sapiens*? Are metabolic and structural similarities between these species enough to ensure successful organ transfer? Is trans-species tissue matching indeed possible? Are breakthroughs in combatting hyperacute rejection of foreign tissue nearly successful enough to begin to speak instead of acute or, even possibly, chronic immunological responses? In turn, can an LVAD adequately pump blood throughout the human system without proving detrimental, dangerous, or fatal for the implanted patient? Do current design parameters enable a prototype to fit a range of body sizes and patients' needs? How inflexible is the system? Is it indeed best to mimic the heart's rhythm as much as possible, or can the continuous flow of blood, without pulse, stalling, or interruption, prove equally (and perhaps even more) effective in patients suffering from organ failure? Should a pig part or a manufactured device be used only as a "bridge" to transplant, or are they trustworthy enough to serve as permanent forms of "destination" therapy?

As these technical concerns demonstrate, experimental science involves significant temporal gymnastics as researchers imagine the futuristic promises of their efforts. Other equally complicated—though often muted—concerns highlight the quandaries and associated scientific responsibilities surrounding human and animal subjects' physical, emotional, and existential suffering, public receptivity to highly experimental procedures, and the short- and long-term consequences of transformative, embodied technologies. What, then, does temporal thinking accomplish? What does it eclipse? How might associated imaginative thinking be understood as a moral enterprise in highly experimental science? Within this chapter, I probe the moral relevance of these sorts of questions in science.

In the introduction to their edited volume *Timely Assets*, Elizabeth Ferry and Mandana Limbert (2008) address the depletion across several domains of various "objects, subjects, people, and ideas," including such diverse categories as oil and mined substances, endangered flora and fauna, and local histories. As they explain, "resources, resource-making, and resource-claiming are entangled with experiences of time" where sometimes "apocalyptic" warnings surface about their future (3–4). Furthermore, concerning "objects and substances produced from 'nature,'"

> Nothing is essentially or self-evidently a resource. Resource-making is a social and political process, and resources are concepts as much as objects or substances. Indeed, to call something a resource is to make certain claims about it, and those claims participate in an ideational system . . . that has a history, perhaps multiple histories. . . . Moreover, particular expressions of this ideational system, what we might call resource imaginations, often have a strongly temporal aspect; they frame the past, present, and future in certain ways; they propose or preclude certain kinds of time reckoning; they inscribe teleologies; and they are imbued with affects of time, such as nostalgia, hope, dread, and spontaneity. (4)

As the range of essays within *Timely Assets* demonstrates, desires to produce, accumulate, and control prized resources are anticipatory acts driven by anxieties over scarcity, not unlike the ideational system that inspires transplant experimentation. In this light, I am especially intrigued by certain "temporal aspects" of scarcity and, most notably, their moral character. As Ferry, Limbert, and their coauthors underscore, the temporal framing of desired resources is not simply about anticipating a future of scarcity but should also involve probing how scarcity itself comes into being—that is, how the ideation of scarcity lays claim to certain histories while neglecting, ignoring, or erasing others. As their volume demonstrates, threats to survival is a theme that pervades discussions of depleted resources, be they oil reserves, ancient coelacanths, prized rhododendrons, or indigenous narratives. This is reflected in the environmentalist's creed, "extinction is forever" (Lowe 2008).

Experimental transplant science reflects similar features, in that widespread concerns for human organ scarcity render xenografting and bioengineering possible and palatable. Nevertheless, whereas Ferry, Limbert, and their coauthors are most interested in attempts to foreground and thus prevent scarcity and extinction, the scientists whose work interests me accept organ scarcity as an inevitable and thus insurmountable social reality because the supply of fleshy parts of human origin will never match the demand. Whereas preservation becomes a common theme in the ideation of a range of "timely assets," according to Ferry and Limbert, temporal thinking within xeno science and bioengineering respond to impeding threats of scarcity by *redirecting* concerns by way of radically new trajectories that will altogether circumvent demands placed on dwindling supplies of human body parts. Experimental transplant scientists take scarcity as a thing of the past (or strive to make it so) and thus as a sociomedical threat rendered obsolete in the future by their ongoing efforts to generate alternatives. Xenografts and mechanical heart devices are like the solar, wind, and geothermal alternatives to dwindling supplies of "black gold," like species cloning to protected reserves and zoo-based breeding, and like the hybridization and genetic modification of domesticated plants to archived seed vaults. Put another way, xeno and bioengineering experts seek actively to reconfigure transplant medicine so as to ensure future biosecurity through alternative sources. In this sense, their radical alternatives reconfigure biosecurity (Sharp forthcoming) in a newly imagined, post-millennial medical future.

As I demonstrate below, these scientists' endeavors to imagine, anticipate, and legitimate experimental alternatives necessitate a particular sort of temporal thinking, where efforts are focused not on the immediate present but on a distant horizon. This sort of temporal shift informs what Jane Guyer (2007) identifies as "promissory" or "prophetic" thinking, a stance that enables scientists to side-step present realities by focusing instead on imaginative, "prophetic" alternatives. As such, temporalized longing defines the very core of the scientific imagination in experimental transplant work. Furthermore, experimentation becomes a moral project intent on alleviating scarcity and human misery; yet, paradoxically, it also naturalizes the erasure of more troublesome thoughts about scientific failure, alongside the suffering of experimental human and animal subjects. Prized values associated with risk taking, maverick science, "thinking outside the box," and the like foreground certain moral concerns while distancing the scientist from vulnerable patients and expendable lab animals. I must underscore that such practices should not be construed as unethical as understood within a bioethics framework: in fact, all researchers whom I have encountered are meticulous in their attention to patient consent, animal welfare, and palliative clinical and veterinary practices. Rather, what I intend to address here are the histories—and future trajectories—of quotidian behaviors that expose ethics in the making. In a sense, one might well think of scientific involvement as incorporating what novelist China Miéville (2009) provocatively identifies in radically different quarters as the cultivated paired practices of "seeing" and "unseeing." In their own ways, and in their own particularized domains, xeno scientists and bioengineers privilege certain key understandings of bodies, devices, and people while erasing from view—and consciousness—conflicting imagery, ideas, and sentiments that are, nevertheless, in plain sight (see Bille et al. 2010).

TEMPORAL LONGING

Of particular significance here is the temporal nature of moral reasoning. When framed as such, moral concerns, convictions, frameworks, and the possibility for consensus must inevitably be understood as flexible, evolving, and mutable. From a policy standpoint (or even from within a bioethics framework), such a position can prove maddening because values appear slippery or situational. Such an approach likewise presents profound ethnographic challenges. It is, nevertheless, a stance that demands a more deeply nuanced approach to moral thinking than does, say, the consistency of principlism (Beauchamp and Childress 1979) and the ethics of care. My purpose in this chapter is to disentangle the relevance of temporality within experimental science and to track the various ways this relationship affects how xeno scientists and bioengineers imagine the possibilities their respective projects entail. That is, how might long-term involvement with various (even competing) highly experimental ideas, procedures, and devices shape the trajectory of everyday ethics in these expert domains?

Throughout this chapter, I strive to examine temporality as an inescapable moral presence that permeates experimental actions, thoughts, and aspirations. The question, then, is what sorts of realities, or "ideational" premises, undergird the work of experimental scientists who strive to reconfigure the sociomedical process of human organ replacement? Whereas those with whom I have worked would most certainly balk at the idea that their projects are driven by "sentiment," *longing and desire* most certainly inform their efforts. Furthermore, involvement in experimental transplant research requires a rather hefty load of patience: as Roy Calne has emphasized, xeno transplantion "is, and always will be, the future" of transplant research (personal communication, July 2010; see also Calne 2005), a phrasing that has emerged as a mantra of sorts throughout the field. Indeed, many xeno scientists whom I have interviewed assume that they will not live long enough to witness the successful implantation of porcine organs in humans. In essence, *temporality* is inescapable for them. Within bioengineering, in contrast, where a range of devices are now increasingly employed clinically, temporal longing assumes different trajectories, encompassing seemingly unending efforts to "perfect" or further "enhance" the design, function, and capabilities or capacities of implants.

In many ways, temporal open-endedness emerges as inevitable within experimental science, because outcomes are unknown. Yet the vagueness of the future is understood differently within bioengineering and xeno science, their concerns framed by distinct temporal registers. The inventive process so central to bioengineering insists on an ever-shifting future horizon by the mere fact that every design is open to further refinement. This sense of the infinite rests at the very core of tinkering.[1] Within xeno, however, one encounters the inescapable tension that research objectives might never be realized because of the complexities of transspecies immune responses and public resistance to hybridity. Perceptions of temporal open-endedness, then, are celebratory in bioengineering and laced with anxiety in xeno science, enabling a sense of moral virtue in the former and apprehension in the latter.

In addition, experimental work is extraordinarily difficult to sustain without access to reliable funding sources. As I demonstrate below, the market itself affects moral thinking, actions, and outcomes in these two domains of science, and this is especially evident when venture capital comes into play. Bioengineering has proved far more successful in sustaining investors' interests, and the field more broadly speaking has a much longer history of involvement in the marketplace. By comparison, xeno experts have struggled to woo and sustain the interest of investors, who withdraw support when hopeful outcomes appear too sluggish for their tastes. Xeno science suffers from the added burden of public perceptions of their efforts as unethical acts of scientific hubris, and in response they now engage in "translation" efforts to persuade nonspecialists outside their respective fields to understand and embrace their work as morally transformative acts of great social worth.

A key question, then, is how to track temporal thinking in science. In this regard, Guyer's (2007) essay "Prophecy and the Near Future" provides a detailed roadmap. Writing of the postmodern turn in anthropology, Guyer exposes what she perceives as an "evacuation" or "evaporation of the near future" as theorists have become increasingly entrenched in discussions of more remote temporal frames. As she explains, the "shift in temporal framing" involves "a double move, toward very short and very long sightedness, with a symmetrical evacuation of the near past and the near future" (410). In such contexts, Guyer asserts, "ultimate origins and distant horizons were both reinvigorated, whereas what fell between them was attenuating into airy thinness, on both 'sides' (past and future) of the 'reduction to the present'" (410, after Jameson 2002, 707, 709). Guyer draws initially on what she perceives as detrimental temporal shifts in anthropology, her analysis informed by overlapping domains of "macroeconomic, evangelical, and punctuated time" (409). Her provocative insights likewise offer an intriguing approach to temporalized, moral thinking in experimental transplant science.

As I argue extensively elsewhere (Sharp 2011c), xeno scientists' efforts are focused unquestionably on the *longue durée*, a "prophetic" stance (Guyer 2007) driven by scientific desires that celebrate achievements during a golden era of key research events that spanned the 1960s to 1990s. This "punctuated time" in turn enables an idealization of a distant future where the seamless integration of porcine parts and human bodies becomes possible. Such a stance necessitates, in Guyer's terms, the "evacuation" and thus the erasure of both the not-so-distant past and the imminent future, two temporal phases that frame present efforts and that, within xeno science, are marred by unending failure in the form of hyper-accute graft rejection, patient suffering, inevitable death, and the possibly futile sacrifice of sentient and, sometimes, large numbers of animals. By leveraging temporal framing in the *longue durée*, hope remains focused on an unknown horizon. In this sense, xeno scientists legitimate a field currently plagued by failure, such that xenografts emerge as viable and moral alternatives to allografting in the distant future (Sharp 2011c). Temporal framing likewise affects one's moral vision within xeno science: when future hopes displace current failures, the latter, rendered less significant, evaporates from view. To prophesize in xeno science means to anticipate outcomes that one has yet to witness, postulating that their associated promises and possibilities are worthwhile pursuits with realistic results. Mishaps, misguided assumptions, and dead ends are refunneled into and inform a scientific logic that insists one learn from mistakes and that a return to the drawing board is part and parcel of experimental inquiry. At each step, one anticipates the possibility of multiple outcomes or futures, and the hope that this inspires is framed, without question, as a moral pursuit. Again, as I argue in more detail elsewhere (Sharp 2011c), stylized temporal thinking in xeno science "foregrounds heroics over hubris, ingenuity over failure, and morality over the marketplace" (45).

Bioengineering likewise relies on temporal thinking, but it demonstrates a different prophetic mode. Differences hinge in part on the nature of involved technologies: for instance, public response (such as reticence, fear, or wonder) can be radically different when faced with inert mechanical gadgetry versus fleshy parts derived from sacrificed, sentient creatures (Sharp 2007). Yet temporal framing also takes its toll, affected by the stark reality that LVAD and TAH devices are now implanted with increasing frequency in patients throughout the United States and Europe. These implants are touted by the mainstream press as major breakthroughs in contemporary medicine, and they regularly win awards for their functional capabilities alongside their sleekness in design (Sharp 2009, 2011b). There is unquestionably a moral aesthetic (Nicewonger 2011; Taylor 2011) at work here that one does not encounter in the world of xenografting, where, instead, animals must be humanized—and thus renaturalized in an ideological sense—to captivate the press, medical specialists, public funding sources and private investors, and potential patient-consumers. Yet another factor that distinguishes bioengineering from xeno science is the extent to which the former is embedded within the marketplace.

MARKETING LIFE

Venture capital is by its very nature fickle, and its involvement with experimental science can be precarious and prickly. Within domains of experimental transplant research, inventors' and investors' lives are frequently intertwined, a relationship that disrupts the temporal frame of scientific morality. As detailed above, experimental scientists are focused on the *longue durée*, a stance that facilitates side-stepping the quandaries of the near future; in contrast, investors inevitably desire rapid or "timely" results and profits. Researchers specifically bemoan the temporal dissonance associated with venture capital, where the realities of the science itself might well be conceived of as irrelevant knowledge among those claiming financial involvement with various laboratory efforts. Among bioengineers, the pressure from investors to create products and thus reach a particular endpoint is antithetical to the process of invention, where every device is potentially subject to further tinkering and perfecting. Xeno science, moreover, has been hard hit by the precariousness of investor interest, experiencing swifter retraction of funds than has bioengineering. As investors' enthusiasm wanes, so too does the flow of capital, rendering research vulnerable to the lack of essential support. Investors sometimes make preemptive moves quite suddenly, abandoning a laboratory for competitors whose efforts might appear more promising and, thus, profitable.

The venture capitalist's ethos is clearly exemplified in Maeder and Ross's (2002) assessment in *Red Herring* of the comparative values and risks associated with investing in xeno and bioengineering, where the former comes in at a distant second because it is too "messy" and "fleshy" to compete with the sleek and, seemingly, more predictable outcomes of engineered hardware. The pressure to demonstrate successful outcomes can also generate disturbing consequences within the laboratory itself. As detailed in chapter 2, the unrealistic expectations of outside investors led one xeno firm in the United Kingdom to sacrifice primates in unprecedented numbers in hopes of rapidly generating promising results. Though a harrowing cautionary tale, this remains an exceptional event, and of greater significance to my own work are the more mundane moral actions that characterize quotidian laboratory life. Research, after all, always relies on the flow of capital—be it derived from one's own income, independent investors, federal agencies, the military, pharmaceutical and other corporations, or nonprofit organizations—and associated relationships readily transform research objectives, techniques, procedures, ideas, devices, animals, and patients' bodies into potentially lucrative forms of biocapital.

Tinkering with Biocapital

As Maeder and Ross's assessment suggests, bioengineers have more opportunities to partner with venture capital than do xeno scientists, a practice rooted in the history of engineering itself. Unlike immunology and genetics, for instance, engineers have long drawn distinctions between those involved in "pure" versus "applied" science, the former more firmly focused on academic research, the latter on developing marketable patents, materials, methods, and inventions, processes most often associated with industrial or corporate employment. Among the bioengineers I have encountered who hold academic posts, all are involved in at least one "spin-off"—an offsite firm through which they design, manufacture, and market their devices and ideas.[2] In turn, inventors with corporate and military ties regularly invoke such concepts as the "trade secret" and "proprietary knowledge" during question-and-answer periods at professional conferences when they are asked about various details in design, or when their peers probe their data and findings.[3] In fact, when I request interviews with bioengineers, I have learned to preface these with assurances that I am not interested in the specific details of device design and, further, that I will not report to others what I see. This approach strikes xeno experts as unnecessary and even humorous. When I spoke of this with Peter Grimaldi, for instance, he responded sardonically by saying "that's absurd—we're all stuck together in the same deep hole!" During personalized tours of bioengineers' labs, it is not uncommon for my guide to check first to see if anyone within is actively involved in device manufacture before I am invited to enter a room or peer through an observation window. Xeno experts instead practice extreme caution so as to prevent visitors from viewing laboratory animals (and especially primates), as dictated by strict regulatory protocols, or transmitting pathogens to them.

In these ways, proprietary knowledge within bioengineering marks the boundaries of a particular sort of black box in experimental science: regardless of how colleagues rephrase queries intended to fine-tune their own understandings of a presentation, the speaker might well provide only partial or even elusive answers. Such firewall tactics are driven by the lucrative quality of bioengineered body parts. One nevertheless encounters a proliferation of devices across different laboratories and firms whose respective designs may well approximate those of competitors while remaining distinct enough to avoid patent disputes. I conjecture that such practices circumscribe the boundaries of moral communities and may well account for the somewhat obsessive propensity among bioengineers to assert genealogical ties, because trade secrets are best shared only among members of one's own clan.

When I visit the bioengineering labs of offsite firms, corporate production sites, and clinically based heart institutes, there is inevitably a visible archive of artifacts housed within a display case set in public space, such as a hall or entryway. Engineers are, it seems, collectors of a specialized sort, and their archives typically track the design progress of VADs, TAHs, and other heart devices over three decades or more. Sometimes these consist merely of a shelf where an array of hardware is stored in plain site and readily available to anyone wishing to demonstrate to visitors (be they investors, potential patients, the media, or an inquisitive social scientist) how the technology has changed over time. In one instance, such a case contained nearly fifty different heart valves of mechanical, porcine, and bovine origins, representing a host of firms and years of manufacture. In other instances, they consisted of much larger and carefully curated displays that took up an entire glassed-in wall in a hospital, with sample devices assembled from an engineer's private collection (see figure 15). Such displayed artifacts mark the collector's long-term involvement in the field, complemented by additional pieces donated

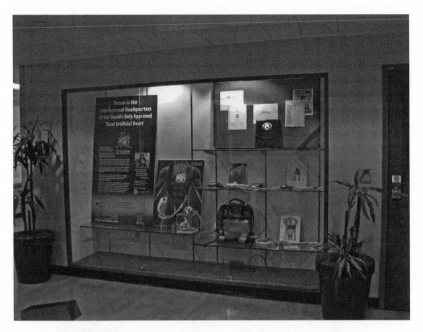

Figure 15. Display case of various heart devices located outside the Artificial Heart Center at the University of Arizona Medical Center in Tucson. The headline text on the poster to the far left reads: "Tucson is the International Headquarters of the World's Only Approved Total Artificial Heart." (Photo by author, June 2012, used with the permission of the University of Arizona Medical Center, Tucson.)

by colleagues working elsewhere for various industries. Still other devices may well have been "explanted" or "autopsied" from individual patients' bodies. Typically, these explanted devices are carefully labeled and mounted on plaques reminiscent of trophies, serving to highlight genealogical linkages among experts and internationally known patients from the past (such as Barney Clark and William Schroeder) or local patient-heroes of bygone days whose surgeries were milestones in the field (as exemplified by young Willie Maskiell in Tucson; see figure 16). One cannot help but notice, too, the shifts over time of device size and morphology: one might find it difficult to imagine how the early pumps could ever have fit within the rib cage of any human being; in other instances, one puzzles over how a device as small as, say, a pair of fingers could indeed pump blood throughout an entire body. As such, these archives serve to demonstrate scientific prowess, ingenuity, and technological refinement over time.

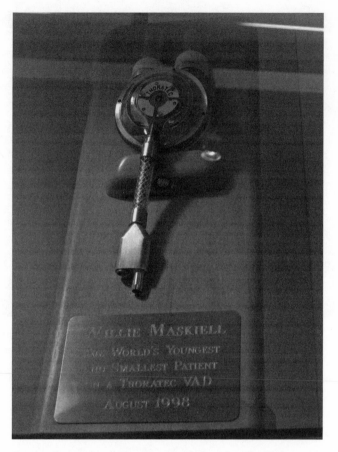

Figure 16. Closeup of upper left corner of display case in figure 15 showing a
Thoratec excorporeal VAD that supported a pediatric patient. The text reads:
"Willie Maskiell / The World's Youngest and Smallest Patient With a Thoratec VAD
/ August 1998." (Photo by author, June 2012, used with the permission of the
University of Arizona Medical Center, Tucson.)

"Commons" Sense

Although xeno experts most certainly court investors, and several have
established "spin-off" companies or now work in the private sector for pharmaceutical and other corporations, their moral frame of reference where
biocapital is concerned stands in stark contrast to that exemplified by many
bioengineers. Among the more striking differences is an emergent commons, marked by a nonproprietary handling or open sharing of specially

bred animals. One Australian researcher described the origin of such practices to me in a 2008 interview as follows: " When [the] Pharma . . . companies got involved [in the 1990s], I couldn't believe how much money there was early on, it was bloody awful—no one would talk to anyone. [They were] very secretive about their work [while] competing for the same pots of money. Then they [Pharma] withdrew [their funding], and xeno went academic. So that's who's left—and they're nicer now. There are patents, but it is more academic now. When they're closer to money, people change."

Rather than regarding specialized strains of hybrid or humanized pigs in proprietary terms, I have encountered several instances where private, commercial labs and their associated farms willingly share animal stock with others. In other words, xeno experts more readily elide the categories of competitor and colleague, shouldering together the challenges associated with ever-shrinking research funds and the difficulties in creating, sustaining, or acquiring specialized, hybrid animals. Such animals figure prominently as scarce resources within an emergent moral economy shaped by financial and regulatory hardships. Xeno scientists frequently cite the retraction of funding sources as the impetus. Whereas a decade ago U.S.-based researchers, for instance, could rely on funding streams from federal agencies and pharmaceutical corporations, caution has displaced former widespread enthusiasm. Various xeno experts now devote their time (and animals) to other more easily funded pursuits, with xeno defining a modest sideline activity. In other words, the current scarcity of resources plays a significant role in the ad hoc sharing of those resources, as xeno experts hold out and wait for future scientific breakthroughs and associated economic windfalls.

The moral underpinnings of this approach is illustrated by the following exchange with Lance Drummond, a highly respected senior xeno scientist in his seventies who hails from the United Kingdom and has worked in several countries over the course of his career. Drummond has spent the past decade developing a strain of humanized pigs at a research center and associated farm in the United States:

LS: When do you think [whole organ transfers] will be possible?

LD: [Chuckling] For the last twenty-five years I've been saying "in five years." . . . [A colleague's team, based in the United States,] has been talking to the FDA, and they're moving to clinical trials involving islet cells. It's an ordinary wild type pig with immuno-suppressant drugs. [If they can demonstrate effectiveness here,] then they'll say they need to go and genetically modify pigs. We'll give them the pigs.

LS: I'm surprised by the level of cooperation—[xeno experts] seem to share pigs with each other, and give them to other researchers who need them. [In contrast, bioengineers] are protective of trade secrets. Why the difference?

LD: But we get something out of it. It will benefit [our] company—[later] we can sell the pigs and then we get some of the credit if it works. We're actively giving out a lot of pigs. To NIH [National Institutes of Health], to [researchers in Europe]. There are two reasons we're doing this: [first], we want to see the whole field progress—there's too much to do and too much in the way of expenses. To get to the clinic—I'm old and I've been doing this for twenty-five years. [And, second,] commercial: if someone is going to test your pigs you get a lot of reward out of it.

Courting Venture Capital

In contrast, senior bioengineers now devote much attention to professional-izing younger members in their field, honing their skills in order to be successful and savvy in the marketplace. This is most evident in the fact that, within the past five years or so, the annual programs of associated conferences have increasingly included fee-based luncheon workshops on how to package and market one's products. These sessions require advanced registration and often have long waiting lists (and, sometimes, a crowd of late comers who have paid for "standing room only" and listen intently while crammed into the back of the room or even spill out the door into the adjoining corridor). Typically, these workshops are run by bioengineers who have successfully marketed devices, alongside venture capitalists who specialize in medical gadgetry and who are always on the lookout for new ideas. In light of such developments, graduate students in particular speak frankly of the moral struggles they face when determining their professional trajectory. Among the more pronounced concerns involves whether or not to accept military funding. Artificial organs are understood in some quarters as yet another form of high-tech body prosthetic and, like myoelectric limbs, are of interest to the U.S. army and the like. The Defense Advanced Research Projects Agency (DARPA) of the U.S. Department of Defense[4] invested fairly heavily in VADs and other associated devices throughout the 1990s, and many students' academic supervisors may well have begun their careers as military engineers (see Sharp 2011b). Bioengineers must thus weigh the morality of military needs against their desire to advance their own research, and some gravitate toward heart devices in part because they view such work as irrelevant to combat needs. As Kay Blalock explained to me, "People will always go where there's money. There has been a huge increase in funding in the past twenty years [in bioengineering]. . . . If you don't want to do the military—it's really challenging. . . . I talked to someone over lunch today who is in industry who said just that—'I know that weapons are necessary, but that doesn't mean I have to make them,' and so he went into biotech."

A more common concern involves whether or not to pursue employment in the private sector. Graduate students often worry that they will drift too far from the engagement that intellectual challenges entail, losing touch with "pure" scientific pursuits that characterize university-based training. In this sense, the lucrative promises of industrial employment are perceived as a corrupting force. Nevertheless, they also understand engineering to be a pragmatically oriented field, and many of their mentors can claim former experience and training in both military and industrial contexts. Commercial enterprises enable them to participate in what might well turn into a fast-paced involvement in device innovation. Those fortunate enough to become involved in small and, later, successful start-up companies express a joyful enthusiasm for the breakthroughs their efforts entail.

Such an approach remains completely foreign to the world of xeno science. Instead—and as I detail below—xeno scientists are deeply involved in efforts to render their research more palatable to a suspicious public through activities they identify as "translational" work. Nevertheless, within each of these competing contexts, potentially lucrative biocapital (Franklin and Lock 2003; Sunder Rajan 2006) entails several things: innovative ideas, artificial devices, genetically altered animals, and implanted human bodies.

Associated activities exemplify the moral underpinnings of respective idea-tional systems where "nostalgia, hope, dread, and spontaneity" (Ferry and Limbert 2008, 4) drive laboratory pursuits and professional trajectories.

The promissory qualities of inventiveness are nevertheless precarious: many a start-up company has gone bust, and senior researchers may have watched a host of efforts fail to win FDA approval or attract a client base. Just as many bioengineers track their personal histories through professional pedigrees, some similarly do so through accounts that string together failed companies (along with associated devices and patients) as a means to ground their life stories in well-known (and, sometimes, notoriously legendary) events. Hendrik Linsdahl, a bioengineer whose eclectic training informs a strongly unconventional moral streak, put it thus during an interview: "Anyone involved in the marketing process will tell you there's always a bal-ance over promise and exaggeration." In turn, as Simon Fletcher asserts, promissory science readily incorporates the improbable and impossible:

SF: In 1975 I went out to work with Kolff [in Utah]. Just to see a whole team [at work] was amazing. They were working on the artificial heart. But I saw some things there that weren't real. . . . They had a *wearable* artificial kidney. The problem was [they wanted it] out on the market, but they had over-hyped it. They had funding from [a major private medical foundation] in New York. But you still had to hook it up to a large device. To get it up that way [i.e. promote it]—it was not really—[you see,] because it had been over-hyped it never got funded.

LS: What about competition among experts? In some instances I encounter open hostility.

SF: All of this is [really about] collaboration. You don't take someone's idea and then make it and not cite others. It's not the "DeBakey" heart but it's called that [because DeBakey] did this [i.e., insisted it bear his name]. [But] these [individual] efforts usually fail. Those who work entirely on their own never get out of the box. . . . A little competition is a good thing.

The marketing of ideas, techniques, and devices is not, however, a uni-versal practice within bioengineering, and controversies over proprietary knowledge and ownership extend back to the early years of artificial organ design. This is evident in the moral framework espoused by Willem Kolff. As historian Steven Peitzman explains, Kolff was "an emblematic figure in twentieth-century medicine. His way of moving medicine forward was through technology" (quoted in Brown 2009). Yet Kolff never sought to patent his dialyzer; as he himself stated, "At that time, it was thought to be unethical for a doctor to make any money on an invention" (also quoted in Brown 2009). Those trained under Kolff often remind me that he preferred that heart devices developed in his labs bear the names of graduate students who supervised these projects, an approach (and, perhaps, incentive) that simultaneously granted credit where due while inadvertently undermining the notion of research as a cooperative venture. (Ironically, this sometimes led to the development of successful patents.) Kolff's assigning credit to individuals in fact runs contrary to the dominant ethos of contemporary laboratory science. Again, in the words of Fletcher, a highly decorated inventor who holds a host of patents, "Those who work entirely on their own never get out of the box."

TRANSLATING SCIENCE IN A WORLD OF UNCERTAINTY

The patenting of life is an increasingly common strategy within the world of biotech (De Witte and Ten Have 1997; Pompidou 1995; Raines 1991; Skloot 2010), and xeno researchers are hardly immune to this. Nevertheless, xeno researchers are far less interested in proprietary practices than they are in managing public perceptions of the promises and dangers of their work. Bioengineering is frequently showered with accolades for artificial organ design, often winning prizes for "best design" or "innovation of the year" (see Hamilton 2001; SyncardiaSystems 2012; VAD for Kids Is Honored 2012). In contrast, xeno science defines a prime target for animal activists and GMO (genetically modified organism) opponents whose accusations of "immoral" and "monster" science have led to moratoriums on xeno research at various times in the United States, the United Kingdom, and Australia. These obstructionist moves stymie scientists' efforts to move their research from the lab to the clinic; more drastic measures can bring the research itself to a complete and utter halt. In the United States, for example, some legislators have sought to regulate or ban the production of human/animal hybrids, as exemplified by Arizona's HB 2652, passed in 2010 (see New AZ Law 2010). In addition, U.S. Senator Sam Brownback of Kansas has mounted ongoing attempts to do the same at the national level.[5] Although not exclusively framed as such, these and other legislative moves have rendered xeno research all the more controversial because the opposition makes misguided claims that the production of human/animal hybrids relies on human embryonic cells and tissues; other lawmakers seem to wish to impose protectionist legislation with the needs of agribusiness within their rural states in mind.[6]

In response, "translational science" has emerged as a buzz-phrase in xeno circles, circulating within this discipline as a new concept associated with the management and legitimation of their work in the public sphere.[7] When I attended an international xeno conference in Europe in 2009, for example, "translational" work was evoked over the course of several days as a newly conceived promissory theme within the field, and three scientists told me spontaneously during interviews that they were engaged in "translational" research in the United States, Europe, and Australia, respectively. It is especially intriguing how xeno experts themselves "translate" the meaning of this term. In its original sense, the phrase was intended to reference what has long been known in science as the movement of experimental breakthroughs "from bench to clinic" (that is, from the laboratory to patient-based practices). Xeno experts certainly use it this way, yet they also apply the phrase quite literally to instances where they seek to "translate" and, thus, "make sense" of their work for a naïve and suspicious public.[8]

An example of this blending of translational meanings surfaced during my discussion in 2009 with xeno expert and immunologist Meredith Kenyon. While negotiating a recent contract with a new academic employer, she had refused to take the offer seriously unless she were granted "full license," as she put it, to develop a "translational" research center, and she had a very complex yet clear vision of what such work would entail. As she explained, "translational" work is about overcoming "insufficient communication" on multiple fronts: encouraging interest among clinicians in the findings of "basic science"; helping a range of parties "understand things we didn't understand before"; and taking advantage of those moments when possibilities for "applied immunology" arise. It is also about developing a sensitivity for the marketability of an idea within the clinic, especially where such efforts require actively "translating" the worth of one's work to an otherwise uninformed public, where the very "language" used may prove pivotal. Kenyon even went so far as to rely on industrial imagery of "vertical and horizontal integration" to drive home her point:

MK: The problem is, whenever an opportunity arises, there isn't always [the recognition that] applied immunobiology [is close at hand]. It's all about translat[ing] basic science—[about] research as basic science. And clinicians don't speak by and large the same language [as we do], or there is a rift between the two. That needs to change. Medicine is more specialized now. There is a lot of pressure on clinicians to perform and earn more money. So old clinical science is very difficult to maintain. It's harder to support centers [because financing is scarce] but the knowledge is much deeper [now]. It's harder for physicians these days, and that's where translational [work matters]. There is insufficient communication between the two; [my job is to demonstrate basic science's] capabilities and what [it] has to offer to clinical areas. It's about . . . vertical and horizontal integration:[9] we need infrastructure—we need access to [clinical] cases.

Through these translational approaches at her new center, Kenyon explained how she intended to promote transparency and public understanding, creating an institutional hybrid of sorts where laboratory work could be intricately intertwined with public policy.[10] Even more interesting was her decision to make a "radical departure" and "fresh start" within the context of her own research efforts. She had devoted the previous fifteen years of her professional life to testing the immunological responses of baboons to porcine organ grafts, but within her new post she intended to work almost exclusively at the cellular level and move into the field of bone marrow transplants. In her words, cellular work—as with pancreatic islet cell research—was "currently understood as the only viable future" for xeno science. For her personally, working at the molecular level ex-vivo and primarily with small rodents was more palatable to her than trying to manage baboons who would ultimately die from hyper-acute porcine graft rejection. When I asked her about employing primates in research, she replied as follows:

> MK: It's simply not tenable to think about using them [because of the realities of a host of trans-species infections]. It's simply not tenable. Many of us have problems using primates. They're *intelligent* animals . . . choosing to use them makes us uncomfortable. I certainly am. Making use of large animals [of any sort], that's something I struggle with. [But] small animals always translate through large animals through nonhuman primates.

It is worth noting, too, that by the late 1990s Kenyon had become heavily involved in drafting policy that ultimately recrafted the ethical parameters of work within her field internationally.

Translational research in xeno reveals an economy of a different sort, where the moral framing of scientific responsibility is weighed down by a prolonged longing to generate viable and safe hybrid forms. The emergence of an animal commons might well be viewed as an act of desperation, where notions of scarcity pervade not only discussions of dwindling supplies in human organs but financing for experimental work as well. I have witnessed, on occasion, marks of desperation surface among xeno researchers from a range of national contexts (Anglophone and non-) in instances where the reliability of research findings is muddied by the simultaneous use of primates for a host of graduate students' projects. As a result of this doubling, tripling, and quadrupling up of invasive procedures on an individual animal, it becomes impossible to know whether one experiment over others generated system-wide immune responses, infections, or death. Labs stretched to the brink sometimes find no other solution when faced with the current predicament of scarce resources. Yet I conclude that xeno science, whose experts generally have neither worked for private, for-profit industries nor engaged much with venture capital, see the commons in pig husbandry, at least, as an innovation in its own right. In essence, the animal commons facilitates a more open approach to sharing and broadening common knowledge than has long been possible in bioengineering circles.

THE CALCULUS OF LIFE AND DEATH

Amid such temporal longings are, of course, ever-present questions of patient survivability. Definitions of survival within clinical contexts are themselves peculiar from a lay point of view: within transplant medicine, a patient might well be described as having had a successful surgery yet die soon afterward during "recovery" in an intensive care unit from "other complications." These might include the failure of other organs, an uncontrolled infection, or ineffective sutures. Moreover, transplant—or, more commonly phrased, graft—"survival" has long been measured in relatively short increments: one year, three years, and five years "out" from surgery. Throughout the course of my earlier work on organ transplantation, especially during the 1990s, few clinicians I encountered dared to address ten-year survival rates because they feared they would find very few patients who were still alive.

Transplant patients remain dependent throughout the remainder of their lives on complex, daily regimens of immunosuppressants and a host of other medications to survive, so much so that it is not unusual for transplant recipients to describe themselves as "drug addicts" and "dope fiends" (much to the consternation of their clinical caretakers). In response, patients, their kin, and medical personnel think readily, freely, and simultaneously within multiple temporal registers: no patients can forget the suffering they endured as they awaited news of an organ match; many speak of living "each day at a time," especially if they continue to suffer from pre-transplant health problems and if they find it difficult to tolerate their anti-rejection medications and the normative effects of chronic graft rejection. All parties who are intimately involved in transplant medicine are always aware of the distant past, the immediate present, and the *longue durée*. They have, after all, suffered intense longing for an appropriate organ match; they worry about how long they might survive post-transplant; and post-transplant desires incorporate hopes that they might accomplish various goals or witness milestones in their loved ones' lives now that they have been granted a new lease on life. The paired themes of survival and suffering always remain in sharp focus, enabling the relentless presence and acute awareness of human vulnerability.

This sort of temporal framing is quite unlike the ways in which patients' experiences are so highly abstracted within experimental domains, a contrast that underscores the paradoxical and uncanny simultaneity of the presence and absence of suffering (Bille et al. 2010). As I have sought to demonstrate throughout this final chapter, temporal thinking assumes very different trajectories in highly experimental domains. Xeno experts, for instance, are especially skittish about the near and present dangers associated with their work as imagined within a contemporary framework, instead idealizing a now-distant golden era onset in the 1960s alongside the intense longing associated with a future whose horizon never fully materializes. Bioengineers understand the passage of time as punctuated in still other ways, because the possibilities of artificial organs have now begun to pay off, so to speak, in various quarters. VADs are used with greater frequency as bridges to transplant in many cardiac units nationally and globally, and talk has increased over the viability of employing these as permanent implants. Recent successes involving a few TAHs likewise facilitate the shifting of attention from a distant to a near future of possibilities. In essence, bioengineering is moving beyond the limitations of prophecy and into the here-and-now of satisfied scientific longing.

Specialists within each discipline nevertheless evince clouded vision where patient subjectivity—not to mention the redefinition of human nature—should matter (Clark 1993, 1999; Fox 1996; Lundin 1999; Papagaroufali 1996; Sharp 2006a, 2009). Few scientists speak of how patients must cope with the inevitable psychic and social transformations that would accompany embodied hybridity, or the vulnerability one experiences knowing that one's life depends on a well-charged battery pack and a machine that simply must not ever seize up or stall. Even more complex, perhaps, than living with leaky or infected entry points for drivelines or the dangers of zoonoses is the calculus of life and death that such radical surgeries necessitate. Although lab-based scientists themselves demonstrate little regard for such questions, (potential) patients think of the risks and dangers of such transformations all the time. Clinicians at work on the front lines think about them, too.

Joseph Massey, an Anglo-American cardiac surgeon in his mid-fifties based at a teaching hospital in the South, offered these insights on the calculus of life and death:

JM: Before we could implant patients with an artificial pump, we had to have a meeting with the insurance CEOs, etc. The data was [*sic*] there for [patient] mortality and quality of life. The insurers only wanted to know, "where is this going to save us money?" [We explained that] the VAD comes down like a liver [in terms of cost; that is, VADs, like liver transplants, are cheaper in the long run than caring for patients in chronic heart or liver failure]. "How are you going to save me money?"—that's what they kept saying. I said, "I don't know—*dead people are cheap.*" One of the most important things for me is quality of life. I still personally think it's worth it— [If I know] I can give him [the patient] a year, [I should do it].

Massey's assertions underscore an urgency to alleviate suffering in clinical contexts, where risky yet increasingly promising technological alternatives necessitate significant capital investment if lives are to be spared. The actuarial values assigned to human beings expose a calculus of life and death that pervades this clinical sphere. Massey is considered a maverick among his peers, a surgeon expertly trained in allografting yet who responds to the futile reliance on scarce organs of human origin by favoring "cutting edge" VAD and other associated technologies. In Massey's view, these cardiac technologies should be employed not simply as temporary bridges but as permanent alternatives to allografting.

EXPERIMENTAL DESIRE

If "dead people are cheap," then experimental innovations transform clinical notions of futility, facilitating in turn the recalculation of life and death in transplant science. When experimental innovation is framed as such, temporal thinking is envisioned as a moral process. In the face of uncertainty, involved researchers must shift their focus from the near and present dangers of their work, evoking the distant future—while simultaneously romanticizing the past—in their efforts to uphold the promissory nature of their work. These temporal challenges are only further complicated by the possibility of failure, an inescapable risk that currently is especially pronounced in xeno research. As scientists focus their efforts on distant (and shifting) horizons, experimental efforts offer evidence of the prophetic nature of science, where paired promises and perils frame the boundaries of moral thinking.

Bioengineers and xeno scientists imagine such promises and perils in their own distinct ways. Whereas tinkering bioengineers appear to work confidently within an open-ended temporal framework, xeno scientists are skittish about a future where the endpoint remains elusive. A shared consequence, though, is the erasure of suffering endured by experimental subjects, set alongside the sociomedical consequences of radical surgeries that might repair but also radically transform bodies. The reconception of experimental devices, procedures, animal genomics, and human bodies into lucrative forms of biocapital only further accentuates the multilayered abstraction of suffering. Within these two competing experimental domains, desires facilitate the rise of proprietary science in one, and a determination to translate the meaning of uncertainty and danger in the other. Together these responses inform a temporal calculus of life and death, exposing the vagaries of experimental failure, longing, and hope.

Conclusion

The Moral Parameters of Virtuous Science

In April 2012, the Canadian government brought to a halt the paired efforts of Ontario Pork (a conglomeration of hog farmers) and the University of Guelph, who together had sought to drive to market a new hybrid creation known as the "Enviropig." This oddly named creature was hailed by its producers as a "less polluting pig" because its manure was more environmentally friendly than that of your average hog. The Enviropig had been genetically "altered" or "engineered" through the integration of mouse and *E. coli* bacterium genetic material so that the pig's gut could process phosphorous more effectively and excrete less of this mineral into the ecosystem. As involved parties explained, "phosphorus can contribute to algal blooms and other environmental problems." Genetically altered animals are prohibited, however, from entering the food chain in Canada, and so, in the end, scientists responsible for developing the Enviropig retrieved boar semen for long-term cold storage and then euthanized their herds. Cecil Forsberg, a professor whose work on these transgenic pigs extends back to 1999, acknowledged, "It's time to stop the program until the rest of the world catches up. And it is going to catch up" (Pollack 2012).

Forsberg's assessment exemplifies the temporalized ideation of promissory science as encountered in other quarters, too, throughout *The Transplant Imaginary*: amid the celebratory achievements of so imaginative an enterprise as the Enviropig, the lay public, unlike involved researchers, remains skittish when confronted with the possibilities this hybrid animal embodies, driving Forsberg and his colleagues to bank its promissory reproductive capacities in the hopes of encountering a more receptive public—and regulatory response—in the distant future. Although efforts to develop the Enviropig remain free of the urgency to alleviate scarcity that pervades the realm of organ transplantation, the moral principles and associated conundrums are strikingly similar to those encountered within xeno science and bioengineering. For instance, all three domains regard the remaking of animals for human use to be an intriguing challenge; all three celebrate experimental prowess in science; and all three presume that the remaking of life and the refashioning of bodies together define an intrinsically moral enterprise. The Enviropig bears promise as an ample food supply and decreased environmental degradation. So, too, do xeno and bioengineering promise to alleviate resource scarcity and human suffering through deliberate attempts to merge humans with animal parts or hardware. When framed as such, these three highly experimental domains epitomize both virtuosity and virtue in science.

As I have demonstrated throughout *The Transplant Imaginary*, the blurring of human/animal/mechanical boundaries generates complex moral quandaries for xeno scientists and bioengineers. Within xeno science, one regularly encounters experts who celebrate hybridity. Their laboratory-generated forms of interspeciality nevertheless present clear and present dangers to humankind, undermining the current promissory nature of xeno's pigs. Xenografting emerges as a destabilizing force in a double sense: it challenges the social (and even evolutionary) order, and, through its insistence that the body be repaired with animal parts, it disrupts the integrity of the embodied self. That is, whereas hybridity is celebrated within xeno science, it prompts uncertainty, suspicion, and anxiety when one must imagine harboring parts of disparate origins within one's own body.

If we assume for a moment the stance of activists who oppose these radical forms of embodied transformation, their protests alert us, at the very least, to the social anxieties that monsters embody. A "monster" most certainly signifies abomination and dread; yet as its etymology reveals, it derives from the Latin term *monstrare*, "to display" or "show." As Jeremy Biles (2007) argues, "The monster is that which appears before our eyes as a sign of sorts; it is a demonstration . . . a portent; it heralds something that yet remains unexpected, unforeseeable" (3). As Biles urges us to consider, what, precisely, does the monster "demonstrate"?[1] What are the affective responses? Mary Murray (2011), writing specifically of the "monstrous" qualities of xeno and zoonoses, identifies associated anxieties as follows:

> Monsters are deeply disturbing because of their perceived potential to disrupt both the "internal" order of the psyche and the "external" order of society. The specter of monstrous metamorphosis challenges the Cartesian view of the person as a rational[,] self possessed individual with a unified identity as it also points to the possibility of wider patterns of social relationships and social organization becoming destabilized. . . . In the past, it was believed that monsters lived in remote places. . . . Contemporary imaginings about the monstrous proportions of zoonotic disease have included the destabilization and destruction of social relationships and structures in the public sphere, as they have raised the specter of the monster within. (116, 119–20)

This dialectic of internal/external destabilization instills an uncanny sense of irony, because, as Murray explains, "the more we believe that we can control our bodies the more anxious we may become with evidence of the vulnerability of our bodies" (121). These subjective considerations render *morality* and *virtuousness* suspect where experimental science is concerned, because embodying monstrous nature is especially frightening (see Murray 2011, 121). Xeno, in essence, disrupts the integrity of the body, where the necessity of hybridity insists that the "monster," so to speak, lies within, or becomes part of us, ultimately breaching the boundary between self and other.

Although manifestly more subtle than in xeno science, these troubling dilemmas surface within bioengineering, too. The subtlety springs from the fact that bioengineering profits from widespread social sentiments that mechanical organs are doubly inert. First, because they are constructed exclusively of metals and plastics, they are considered "ethics free," encompassing what Arthur Kleinman (2006) has described as "the magical belief in technological supremacy over life itself" (6; see also DelVecchio Good 2001). As a result, bioengineers more easily escape the scrutiny endured by xeno because the latter culls parts from sentient creatures. In turn, the presumably inert nature of "artificial" parts subsequently informs sociomoral understandings within bioengineering, a domain frequently enveloped by a sense of ethical neutrality, and this defines an altogether different sort of inertness in a form best described, perhaps, as moral myopia. Whereas xeno's ongoing failures consign its efforts nearly exclusively to the laboratory, bioengineers now enjoy the luxury of testing on patients the viability of a range of devices in their efforts to repair and, even, perfect the flaws of the human form. Their tinkering has thus emerged as an inherently moral pursuit, a process that nevertheless facilitates the abstraction of human suffering. As the narratives of a handful of experimental patients reveal, mechanical implants do indeed trouble the boundaries of the self, raising unsettling questions about body wholeness and the silencing of suffering (Rice 2003; Sharp 2009; Wainwright and Wynne 2008).

These scenarios of social danger and patient suffering are further complicated by the necessity of employing animal subjects in both xeno science and bioengineering. Whereas xeno thrusts the utilitarian nature of animals front and center, animals are likewise prized work objects within the competing domain populated by bioengineers. A troublesome reality within xeno science is this discipline's long-term dependency on animals as a source of organs, set alongside the ways that involved scientists so frequently distance themselves from the very creatures on whom they rely. This is especially pronounced where nonhuman primates are concerned, animals frequently classified and named in generic ways (such as "Baboon #17") so as to depersonalize them, whereas pigs, as animals long understood as "purely utilitarian," are nevertheless cuddled and coddled at least as long as they remain piglets. Interestingly, intimacy between man and beast is far more pronounced and widespread within bioengineering, where ewes and male calves are handled with care not just during the testing of devices but also long after their deaths, when they are sometimes elevated to a peculiar sort of ancestor, their involvement in science merged with genealogies of scientists and devices that record entangled laboratory lives that span seventy years. These are, without question, very peculiar pedigrees. Whereas xeno's sacrificed animals may leave few traces, those recruited to bioengineering mark the progress of moral science in the making.

Both fields unquestionably insist on the blurring of boundaries between human and animal or machine, and such possibilities frame the promissory nature of each discipline. Each embraces the remaking of nature as a laudatory human and scientific propensity. Each similarly naturalizes the remaking of the human form by grafting onto such bodies parts of either animal or artificial origins. Yet these radical attempts at hybridity trigger certain quandaries. Xeno scientists themselves express widespread reluctance to embody porcine parts, and bioengineers frequently explain that their initial attraction to the field was driven by the self-realization that they are not social creatures—as they put it, "I'm not a people person." Practitioners within each discipline keep their distance from the human and animal suffering and sacrifice their research entails. Although each discipline insists on deliberate—and, for the experimental subject's body, traumatic—surgical interventions, within the laboratory itself these radical, transformative acts are overshadowed by scientists' shared sentiments of conviction and wonder.

THE UNCERTAINTIES OF COMPASSIONATE SCIENCE

Kleinman (2006), writing of vulnerability in medicalized contexts, contends that "dangers and uncertainties are an inescapable dimension of life. In fact . . . they define what it means to be human" (6), and their inevitability instills the importance of striving to live a moral life. For Kleinman, morality is deeply entwined with compassion, a response that arises in one's effort to hold onto that which is most dear, often in the face of "the profound sense of inadequacy and existential fear" (6). Kleinman's reflections provoke us to consider the subjective experiences not merely of willing humans but, I would add, of nonconsenting animals, too, both of which must inevitably bear the consequences of being employed as experimental research subjects (see also Abadie 2010). If we temporalize such experiences, what are the effects of experimental participation in the short and *longue durée*? How might human, chimp, calf, and swine be perceived? How is each transformed? This line of questioning sparks yet another: how might the theme of compassion in the face of "inadequacy and fear" enable us to probe sentimental qualities, ethical frameworks, and moral quandaries as they pertain to experimental scientific practices?

Like Kleinman, I have asked throughout this work how, if bioethics "aspire[s] to universal application" (6), we might probe morality as an everyday experience that informs human action. I ask now, too, how "virtue" might translate as a moral value (25) among researchers' efforts to overcome organ scarcity in transplant medicine. Throughout *The Transplant Imaginary*, I have drawn from ethnographic encounters as a means to identify and decipher individuals' experiences, the personal values embedded in their narratives, and, more broadly, the richness of moral thinking in everyday laboratory life within specialized branches of science (see Kleinman 1999; Lambek 2010; Mol 2002; Mol et al. 2010). Although the theme of compassion has remained on the sidelines, in these final pages I wish to offer a few closing remarks on the significance of this sentiment in experimental science.

At several key junctures of my research, scientists have initiated interviews with proclamations like that voiced by an engineer whom I encountered in mid-2011: as he put it when introducing me to a colleague I had looked forward to meeting, "she really gets it," for which I am forever grateful. On three separate occasions, scientists or clinicians who were at first reluctant to meet with me changed their minds after reading some of my work (see especially Sharp 2009) because, in each case, among their greatest concerns was what one called "the disappearing act of the patient." I reference these moments not in an effort to legitimate my work but to underscore the importance of foregrounding suffering as a key variable of analysis. Similarly, though muted, my interviews within domains of xeno science have taught me that anyone who works with lab animals must face questions about the moral boundaries of their use precisely because researchers must resolve conflicting emotional, social, and scientific sentiments in their efforts to remake animals for science. It is worth noting that, throughout the course of this project, no one whom I sought out turned down an interview request, and, indeed, the only interference I encountered came from an arts administrator and self-appointed gatekeeper who worked as a liaison in a small, specialized hospital between artists-in-residence and surgeons. Put simply, she was skittish about any efforts to probe such themes as "suffering" and "morality" in discussions with fellow employees. Overall, those with whom I met were intrigued by these categories, although they may have struggled at first to find the words to express this. Nevertheless, interviews and less formal encounters regularly led to lively discussions about the meaning of suffering and the relevance of morality to scientific work, especially when researchers readily admitted that they rarely thought of or discussed these themes openly with colleagues. As a result, suffering, morality, and compassion each marked specialized and, even, refined sites of longing and desire within the scientific imagination.

Sometimes interviewees had at least some surgical or bedside experience in hospital settings. The majority of the scientists I interviewed, however, only thought abstractly about how their work might affect broad categories of patients, either during experimental phases of research or even later, if and when their efforts proved successful enough to turn either xenografts or mechanical parts into routine surgical interventions. Of the few who had ventured into hospitals, they typically recounted only post-surgical encounters with patients. In rare instances involving xenotransplants a few decades ago, this generally meant flying in to meet a colleague's patient during recovery. Among bioengineers, the experience is becoming more common; they might well become acquainted with an ambulatory recipient like Peter Houghton whose implanted LVAD or TAH could eventually make hospital discharge a reality.

The few bioengineers I met who have assisted during surgical "fittings" offer a brief glimpse into the possibility that "tinkering" can indeed evidence "care in practice" (Mol et al. 2010). Although these scientists define a minority (and thus, perhaps, are "outliers") within their fields of expertise, they nevertheless expose an intense awareness of and sympathy for the patients whose willing participation as experimental subjects has enabled the advancement of scientific discovery. These experiences foster a different sort of kindredness between scientist and research subject in contexts requiring all involved parties to embrace a moral project that blurs the boundaries between human and animal or machine. Such levels of interest, concern, and compassion are potentialities that inform virtuous acts in science. It is this sort of potentiality that I hope might bloom within these radical branches of experimental science.

In conclusion, I join Brad Weiss (2012) in asking, "What is the appeal of totalities?" Although Weiss's work explores the sentiments of locovores as pork consumers in the United States, his insights prove similarly enlightening to my own work. As he explains, "There is both an aesthetic and ethics at work here as local activists strive for 'a new holism'" (614, 615). If we translate this to encompass quite literally what my students sometimes refer to as a new "wholism"—where human bodies are expected to integrate in seamless fashion implanted parts of foreign origin—we quickly encounter the outer limits of the "what if" promissory qualities of experimental transplant science. Together, xeno scientists and bioengineers seek every day to naturalize technologies that unquestionably disrupt both body and species integrity. If such alternatives can indeed solve the crises wrought by organ scarcity, then renaturalized boundaries, paired with a compassion for suffering, must figure prominently and equally in the moral framing of experimental efforts to tinker with life, significantly broadening the scope of the scientific imagination and its associated desires.

INTRODUCTION

1. See http://www.syncardia.com, consulted Aug. 21, 2011.

2. See http://www.bbc.co.uk/news/health-14363731, consulted Aug. 21, 2011.

3. Ibid.

4. See "Barney Clarke," Scientific American Frontiers, http://www.pbs.org/saf/1104/features/substitute2.htm; see also Fox and Swazey 1992.

5. Still other experimental domains include tissue engineering and reparative nanotechnologies. I have excluded these from this study because prototypes have yet to be realized: although impressive strides have been made in the regeneration of viable tubular tissues (most notably the bladder, trachea, and vagina), whole organs are currently far too complicated in structure and function (see Atala 2005). Nanotechnologies, in turn, perhaps define the most extreme example of imaginative thinking in transplant medicine, where discussions inevitably begin with the phrase "What if we could. . . ."

6. As will become clear below, specialists from a range of fields use "ethics" and "morals" interchangeably. For the sake of clarity, throughout this book I restrict my use of "ethics" to reference codified categories claimed as the purview of formalized bioethics; in contrast, within the context of my own research, I am most interested in the broader category of "morals" (or morality) and thus the far less formalized and, frequently, more highly subjective processes associated with moral thinking in science. In those instances where other authors conflate ethics and morals, I will make this clear in the text.

7. For an intriguing study of the less formal aspects of IRB evaluations, see Stark 2011; on the internationalization of IRB frameworks, see Schrag 2010.

8. For instance, IRB processing at Columbia University, where I am affiliated, requires certification that one has completed several online tutorials, where modules are organized quite explicitly around the Beauchamp and Childress model.

9. Note that, in this context, Banner's use of "ethical" corresponds with the meanings I assign to "moral," as should be clear in the sentence that follows.

10. I employ the expression "organ transfer" to underscore the inseparability of organ donation, retrieval or "harvesting," and transplantation.

11. DelVecchio Good (2001, see 396–97) identifies yet a third interpretative concept, "the clinical narrative" whereby ethnographic attention to patients' experiences reveal "multiple regimes of truth" in science, a concept that is of less concern to me here, although scientists' narratives will most certainly figure prominently throughout this work. Aided by DelVecchio Good's analysis, I wholeheartedly agree with her assessment that there is no singular "truth" at work in experimental contexts.

12. In this instance, the laboratory of Louis Pasteur.

13. Within actor-network theory (ANT) of science studies, as evident in the work of Bruno Latour, John Law, Steve Woolgar, Susan Leigh Star, Annemarie Mol, and others, both humans ("actors") and objects ("actants") are granted agentive qualities. Characterized by a meticulous scrutiny of ongoing interactions of "networks" of the two, ANT offers a quasi-semiotic approach to the production of scientific knowledge and innovation. For an informative introduction, see the collections edited by Law (1986, 1991) as well as Latour 1987; Latour and Woolgar 1979; Mol 2002; and Mol 2008.

14. For compelling examples among moral philosophers who effectively integrate the theory and methods of their discipline and anthropology, see Mol 2002; Mol 2008; and Banner forthcoming.

15. As several authors demonstrate, too, the wonder associated with new technologies can lead involved parties to defer ethical discussions (see DelVecchio Good 2001; DelVecchio Good et al. 1999; Koenig 1988; van Kammen 2003). As still others remind us, emergent technologies also inspire celebratory stories and hype, both of which obscure deeper moral issues (see Franklin and Lock 2003; Sunder Rajan 2006, 107–20).

16. Whereas my encounters and informal discussions now number in the hundreds, the most important interview data reported in this work are drawn from seventy formal, extended (and sometimes multiple), open-ended interviews with eleven bioengineers; eight xeno researchers; two geneticists; a primatologist; fourteen animal-care experts, ranging from personnel of university-based swine facilities to caretakers of primates in research labs; three veterinarians; a nationally appointed regulatory overseer of lab animals; an

anatomist who taught me how to dissect a fetal pig; four animal rights activists; six bioethicists; six surgical experts involved in implanting VADs in patients; fours surgeons who had been early advocates of xenografts; four bioartists whose work addressed xeno science or bioengineering; and five patients implanted with a range of heart devices, including VADs, heart valves, and defibulators.

CHAPTER ONE. THE RECONFIGURED BODY OF THE TRANSPLANT IMAGINARY

1. As I detail below, Brodwin's latest research (2013) is equally significant.

2. Much has been written on the ethics of anthropological research itself, although this is not the central concern among those whom I cite here.

3. May and Abraham Edel were a husband and wife team, and each was trained in one of these two disciplines. Their book *Anthropology and Ethics* grew out of their discussions with one another about the meaning of ethics and morality in their respective disciplines. I thank Michael Banner for drawing my attention to this work. It is also discussed in detail by Zigon (2008).

4. My purpose here is not to quibble with the history but to consider what we mean when we speak of morality or moral systems. For a recent comprehensive compendium, see Fassin 2012.

5. Laidlaw (2002, 2010) and Faubion (2011), for instance, are partial to Foucault, whereas Lambek (2003, 2008) often favors Aristotle, among other philosophers.

6. These principles not only shape scientists' activities and research designs but also inform practices concerning patients' rights, especially in reference to informed consent. As Laura Stark (2011) nevertheless demonstrates, IRB panels may evaluate the quality of proposals based on moral judgments that fall well beyond an institutional regulatory framework.

7. As I demonstrate in chapter 2, still other formalized principles guide research involving the use of animals employed for research purposes in the United Kingdom.

8. In an altogether different vein, Veena Das (2012) terms "ordinary ethics" as a means to focus on human frailty and vulnerability. Especially noteworthy is Das's willingness to pay close attention to those instances where individuals act unethically in their treatment of others or where they refrain from doing so. (For a much earlier handling of some of these same themes, see Bellah 1979.) Where this project is concerned, Das's framing is of greater relevance to, say, the experiences of experimental human and animal subjects, a focus that falls outside the scope of my work.

9. Likewise, Das asks: "In what way might one think of the performance of . . . quotidian acts as constituting an 'ordinary ethics'? Are the sorts of descrip-

tions of everyday life I offer not *too* quotidian to qualify as forms of ethical behavior?" (2012, 138). Similar to my framing of the moral imaginary, as derived from Beidelman 1993, DelVecchio Good 2001, Brodwin 2013, and Lambek 2010, Das is especially interested in what she describes as "the imagination of human action and . . . the moral as a dimension of everyday life rather than as a separate" (or, perhaps, even specialized) domain of experience (138).

10. As I describe elsewhere (Sharp 2011b), bioengineers sometimes rely on Vesalius's work to illustrate their own efforts in public venues.

11. For a discussion of the naming of the exceptional animal, see Miller's (2005, 13–28) account of Goldie the pig (alias pig #15502) in a Harvard xeno lab.

12. As described recently by musician Simone Felice, who in June 2010 received a mechanical heart valve, the device's clicking sounds permeate his music. According to an interview on NPR: "On the recordings—I recorded most of them in my barn in the Catskills—I could not for the life of me get the tick out of the recording. . . . I had to put three or four sweaters on, and a ski jacket, and you can still hear it. So we turned up the volume, and at the end of the album, you can hear the heart tick for about 20 seconds" (http://www.npr.org/2012/04/08/150009291/simone-felice-the-solemn-sound-of-a-brush-with-death, Apr. 8, 2012).

13. For a fascinating example of shifting boundaries between humans and animals in laboratory contexts, see Svendsen and Koch forthcoming.

14. For Rose (2007, 29), "somantic ethics" simultaneously encompasses embodied experience, suffering, and biological knowledge and associated interventions.

CHAPTER TWO. HYBRID BODIES AND ANIMAL SCIENCE

1. Here Leach writes of how a young child learns to "determine the initial boundary" of self from other and of the body's boundaries in specific reference to taboos.

2. A fairly rich literature has been generated from within anthropology that addresses the attitudes of potential patients and more general lay public toward xenografting and transspecies genetics. See Cook 2006; Lundin 1999; Lundin and Idvall 2003; Murray 2006, 2007, 2011; Papagaroufali 1996, 1997; Sharp 2011a; and Taussig 2004.

3. For the sake of brevity, from this point forward I will employ the term *primate* to designate those that are nonhuman, except where noted otherwise.

4. As announced in late 2011, the U.S. National Institutes of Health will no longer support research involving chimpanzees (Gorman 2011a, 2011b, 2011c).

5. The use of chimps and monkeys in xeno corresponds in interesting ways with their employment in NASA's space program (see Sharp 2007).

6. It is now widely accepted in many quarters that pigs are highly intelligent creatures. However, the fact that they are also still widely seen as farm animals has slowed the pace at which scientists, regulators, or activists rise to their defense as worthy of protection from laboratory research, a categorization I discuss later in this chapter.

7. My earliest work on xeno extends back to the late 1980s, when I was employed as a research assistant by Margaret Clark (1999); my initial interest had been sparked a bit earlier by the episode in 1984 involving Baby Fae (discussed later in this chapter). Starzl's attempts at baboon-to-human liver transplants coincided with my work on allotransplantation (Sharp 2006b).

8. Interestingly, this approach is not so common in other countries. Also, the widespread use of fetal pigs is relatively new in the United States; scientists in their mid-fifties, for example, tell me they more routinely dissected cats or frogs in their youth. I suspect the rise of industrial swine farming in some countries informs these pedagogical practices as much as it does the altered path of xeno research.

9. Michael Jackson (2002) offers a similar observation in a discussion on intersubjectivity and human-animal relations in xenotransplantation. As he notes, "There is abundant evidence that ritual and intellectual techniques for crossing the boundaries between animal and human domains (shape-shifting, totemism), or between nature and culture (fetishism, anthropomorphism), occur in all societies and at all times" (343).

10. See http://www.geneticsandsociety.rsvp1.com, accessed Dec. 11, 2011. The original Chimera was a monster of significant stature in Greek mythology. It was the offspring of Echidna, the sibling of other monsters, including Cerberus, and, according to some accounts, it was the mother of the Sphinx and Nemean Lion. The Chimera terrorized human populations in Asia Minor and was later slain by Bellerophon, who rode the winged horse Pegasus. Contemporary immunologists have since embraced the term to describe the immunological compatibility of diverse species within a single body. Chimerism is the desired goal within xenotransplantation, and *Chimera* is the title (and symbol) of its international society's most important publication.

11. The same claims are not necessarily true for laboratory technicians and other caretakers.

12. A comical rendition of this aired on National Public Radio on Dec. 24, 2011, during the quiz show "Wait Wait, Don't Tell Me!" when Goodall was asked to comment on a Gary Larson cartoon where a female chimpanzee confronts her mate when she discovers blond hairs from Dr. Goodall in his fur (see http://www.npr.org/2011/09/24/140726396/primatologist-jane-goodall-plays-not-my-job, accessed Jan. 22, 2012). Goodall's ethos of human/animal cohabitation

stands in stark contrast to the approach advocated within anthropology, where efforts to track and record human behavior have long necessitated immersion through the technique of participant-observation. If we turn again to human/animal cohabitation, Haraway's (2003) work on companion species involves exclusively purebred and extraordinarily well-trained canines, creatures who share little if anything in common with either Goodall's wild chimps or the lab-bound animals employed in xeno research.

13. As xeno researchers often tell me, animal welfare in the lab is paramount because healthy animals generate the best data.

14. One need only peruse order catalogues of such animal suppliers as the Jackson Laboratory of Bar Harbor, Maine, or Harlan Sprague Dawley of Indianapolis, Ind., to encounter a range of such creatures. For a history of the laboratory mouse, see Raines 1991.

15. I wish to thank J. C. Salyer for his insights on this topic.

16. The poignancy of this question is reflected in recent assertions that captive chimps should be considered a distinct endangered species (see Gorman 2011c).

17. Among the more poignant stories I have encountered that illustrate this was one told to me by a former research assistant who had applied for a laboratory job where rats were used in research. She was raised as a Buddhist, and during the final interview she was asked if she would be able to sacrifice (that is, kill) animals (she said she was not sure). She was then taken into a room and shown a guillotine device that was promptly used on an expendable rat. She told them that, after observing this, she knew she could not engage in this practice, and she assumed she had lost the job. In the end, she was hired and was told that others would assume this duty and, further, that the euthanizing of animals was always an option and not a requirement. Lab technicians based in the United Kingdom recounted similar stories during interviews I conducted with them there in 2010.

18. The same might be said for humans engaged in clinical trials (see Abadie 2010).

19. See the volumes for Sept. 16, 1935, and June 13, 1938. The second featured Carrel alongside Charles Lindbergh, with whom he designed a heart pump. As will become clear in a subsequent chapter, Carrel is considered a founder not only within xeno science but within bioengineering as well.

20. See, e.g., a letter dated Dec. 21, 1912, written from Lyon, France, by A. Carrel to Dr. Flexner at Rockefeller University, summary from May 8, 1929, on "the Mousery" (Rockefeller Foundation Archives, Rockefeller Archive Center, Sleepy Holly, N.Y., box 450, C232 "Faculty," Alexis Carrel box 1, folder (2) 1906–1916 and folder for 1923–1929).

21. It was not until 1944 that Sir Peter Medawar, a British zoologist, determined that graft rejection was based on immunological responses. (He won the Nobel Prize in 1960 for his theory of acquired immunological intolerance.) A decade later, in 1954, the first successful human-to-human kidney transplant, which involved identical twins, occurred in Boston, Mass. (Cooper 2007).

22. Some experiments in retrospect seem positively bizarre. Among the most noteworthy are Serge Voronoff's (1925) widely applauded efforts in France that involved grafting chimpanzee and baboon thyroid and testicular tissue to older men with the promise of rejuvenating lost virility, essentially xenografting's answer to the pre-Viagra age.

23. I have written of this elsewhere (Sharp 2006a, 2011a, 2011c). For detailed histories, see Auchincloss Jr. 1988; Cooper and Lanza 2000; and Deschamps et al. 2005.

24. A common refrain used by xeno (as well as bioengineering) researchers is the notion of the "maverick," someone whose risk-taking behavior defies current rules (or even regulations) yet who might well make significant strides in the field. Sometimes this distinction is drawn along generational lines. During an interview with me in 2008, an Australian transplant surgeon and researcher in his mid-fifties, when asked to comment on the baboon-to-human liver transfers attempted by Thomas Starzl in the 1990s (see below), put it thus: "Tom was from the old school, so he just did it . . . in the 1960s and 1970s, the 1980s, these guys just did things. In the modern day, I count that as unethical. . . . [Still,] sometimes you need a maverick. You need a few circumstances where you'll take the risk."

25. David Cooper has proved especially determined to uncover details of xeno's history, publishing descriptions as well as exceptionally helpful charts detailing the type of animal used, circumstances, and surgical outcomes. For instance, he provides details for ten xeno heart transplants that were either orthotopic (where the organ is implanted within the body and replaces the ailing organ) or heterotopic (the graft is placed beside or near the ailing organ). Organs were derived from chimps, baboons, pigs, and, in one instance, a sheep (Cooper et al. 2000, 1129 [chart]). See also Cooper 2007; Cooper et al. 2002; Cooper and Lanza 2000; and Deschamps et al. 2005.

26. James Hardy performed the first human lung transplant in 1963 and the first chimp xeno heart transplant in 1964, both in Mississippi. Also in 1963, Claude Hitchcock transplanted a baboon kidney in a human patient in Minneapolis. Keith Reemtsma, originally based at Tulane University in New Orleans, Louisiana, and later at Columbia University in New York City, transplanted a chimpanzee kidney in a woman in 1964 who survived nine months with her xenograft; he performed another five similar surgeries and subsequently conducted foundational research on pancreatic islet cells. Thomas Starzl has long

been regarded as a leader in kidney, liver, and xeno transplants in the United States, with much of his often highly experimental work based in Colorado and, later, in Pittsburgh. Denton Cooley is best known for having implanted the first total artificial heart in a human patient in Texas in 1969. (See Altman 2000; Auchincloss Jr. 1988; BBC 1999; Deschamps et al. 2005; Fitzpatrick 2009; Lederer 2008; Starzl 1992.)

27. Xeno experts still puzzle over why these patients survived as long as they did; both nevertheless struggled with significant health problems throughout the remainder of their post-surgical lives.

28. Three other xeno surgeries (for which few data exist) were attempted between 1992 and 1996. One involved a female patient in Los Angeles who received a pig liver as a temporary "bridge" to allotransplantation (details of the case were not published until 1996). The other two were pig heart transplants in patients in India and Poland; those patients survived between thirty-four hours and seven days. The Indian physician was arrested and charged with violating his country's Human Organ Transplantation Act of 1994 (Deschamps et al. 2005).

29. These restrictions are no longer imposed with any regularity as exclusionary criteria for allografts.

30. The name of this group is a pseudonym, as are those of other organizations and individuals described or cited within this and other chapters. Original names have been preserved only in those instances where individual or organizational identities are linked to their published sources or news reporting.

31. See Campaign for Responsible Transplantation; http://www.crt-online.org, accessed Sept. 22, 2012.

32. One need only consider the research activities that generated Dolly the Sheep to understand the magnitude of relevant research in the United Kingdom (see Franklin 2003, 2007).

33. The Three R's are (and here I quote directly from the regulatory web page, http://www.understandinganimalresearch.org.UK/about_research/animal_welfare_and_the_three_rs, "Understanding Animal Welfare," accessed July 29, 2010):

+ Replace the use of animals with alternative techniques, or avoid the use of animals altogether.
+ Reduce the number of animals used to a minimum, to obtain information from fewer animals or more information from the same number of animals.
+ Refine the way experiments are carried out, to make sure animals suffer as little as possible. This includes better housing and improvements to procedures which minimise pain and suffering and/or improve animal welfare.

This approach dates back to a seminal paper written in the 1960s, although researchers and veterinarians often explained in interviews that they typically learned of this approach once they were employed in laboratories; it was not included in the curriculum during their training. A more recent approach passed in 2006 in the United Kingdom involves what is known as the "Five Freedoms." They consist of the following (I quote directly from the Farm Animal Welfare Council website, http://www.fawc.org.UK/freedoms.htm, accessed July 29, 2010):

> The welfare of an animal includes its physical and mental state and we consider that good animal welfare implies both fitness and a sense of well-being. Any animal kept by man, must at least be protected from unnecessary suffering.
>
> We believe that an animal's welfare, whether on farm, in transit, at market or at a place of slaughter should be considered in terms of 'five freedoms'. These freedoms define ideal states rather than standards for acceptable welfare. They form a logical and comprehensive framework for analysis of welfare within any system together with the steps and compromises necessary to safeguard and improve welfare within the proper constraints of an effective livestock industry.
>
> 1. *Freedom from Hunger and Thirst*—by ready access to fresh water and a diet to maintain full health and vigour.
> 2. *Freedom from Discomfort*—by providing an appropriate environment including shelter and a comfortable resting area.
> 3. *Freedom from Pain, Injury or Disease*—by prevention or rapid diagnosis and treatment.
> 4. *Freedom to Express Normal Behaviour*—by providing sufficient space, proper facilities and company of the animal's own kind.
> 5. *Freedom from Fear and Distress*—by ensuring conditions and treatment which avoid mental suffering.

34. The Nuffield Council on Bioethics was founded by the Nuffield Foundation in 1991. It is an independent entity currently funded additionally by the Wellcome Trust and the Medical Research Council in the United Kingdom (see http://www.nuffieldbioethics.org, accessed Jan. 15, 2012).

35. Within the United Kingdom, New Zealand, and Australia, bioethical concerns are often fielded in public arenas through the formation of "working parties," ad hoc committees that seek out lay opinions on topics that specialists (including bioethicists and others) believe are of concern to—or affect—society at large. Within Australia, for instance, several bioethicists and xeno experts formed such a party, posting notices in national and regional newspapers (and through other media venues) to encourage anyone interested in them to attend public discussions set up around the country. From this ensued a set of recommendations for how best to proceed with xeno in that country. No such approach is employed in the United States; instead, as Margaret Lock (2002) has argued, such issues are considered the exclusive purview of experts.

36. Kennedy was originally a member of the Nuffield Council's committee.

37. Nuffield members were encouraged by Tim Ingold, an anthropologist long known for his work on human/animal relations (see Ingold 1980), to reassess what values informed their preponderance to assign greater worth to some animals over others.

38. As explained by Sarah Franklin (2007, 22), this special sheep was created through somatic cell nuclear transfer, now known as "the Dolly technique."

39. In yet another context, during an interview with me in 2009, a senior xeno researcher who had trained in part under Christiaan Barnard spoke of the ease with which they could obtain captured baboons in South Africa throughout the 1970s because farmers regarded their presence as a nuisance.

40. This is not, in fact, an unusual practice (see Sharp 2012). I have encountered numerous lab personnel—including vets and technicians—who have rescued animals once experiments come to an end. These include rats, rabbits, and, in one instance, several pint-sized monkeys.

41. These surgeries were intended as practice sessions to document that the surgery was possible for a transplant team to perform.

42. This approach stands in stark contrast to how bioengineers work, where public presentations are often truncated because of a desire to protect trade secrets. I offer a detailed comparative discussion of these practices in chapter 4.

43. Interestingly, efforts were under way to designate this island as a bird sanctuary, and feral pigs were considered pests that needed to be eliminated. Cellcraft acquired permission to obtain enough pigs to start two separate, isolated breeding facilities.

44. Immunosuppressants (often paired with steroids) must be taken daily and in hefty doses to stave off graft rejection. A common understanding is that transplant recipients are chronically ill (evident in their need for daily medications and because they are always in a state of rejecting their transplanted organs—and, as recipients themselves emphasize, because these very medications make them feel ill much of the time). The side effects of these drug regimens include indigestion, hirsuitism, swollen facial tissue that generates what is known as a "moon face," persistent acne, osteoporosis, and, even more significantly, unusual cancers. Medications are also typically nephrotoxic and hepatotoxic over time such that, ironically, the very medications designed to stave off rejection may in fact destroy the organ (or other healthy ones) over time. All this, alongside the regular, grueling tests (such as painful organ bioposies) designed to insure a transplanted organ is still a relatively healthy one, can make it difficult to witness presumed recovery in patients and especially children after transplantation. Although only anecdotal, during the 1990s in particular, I had the distinct impression that children with transplants of that era appeared to experience stunted growth as well (something that struck me at the time as one of

transplant's dirty little secrets because no professionals claimed to see what I did; parents and other patients, however, were equally concerned about this).

45. Whereas animal activists berate and expose scientists for exploiting and harming laboratory animals, lab researchers themselves might consider the withdrawal of animals from laboratories—alongside prohibitions on their use—as intrinsically immoral, because knowledge gleaned from working on a handful to a few hundred animals could ostensibly improve or save a multitude of human lives. Such actions do not stand as the lesser of two evils; rather, they are a hallmark of morality in science. In a 2011 *New York Times* article, for instance, which explored whether the use of laboratory chimpanzees should persist in the United States, John VandeBerg, director of the Southwest National Primate Research Center in San Antonio, Texas, explained that "stopping research with chimps would be a threat to human lives" because "[a]ny reduction in the rate of development of drugs for these diseases [specifically, hepatitis B and C] will mean hundreds of thousands of people, really millions of people, dying because it would be years of delay" (Gorman 2011a, D4). As illustrated so succinctly here, animals are valued within science for their utilitarian qualities, and their use figures centrally in the moral drive to advance knowledge and stave off widespread human suffering.

46. For a detailed account of the origins of swine husbandry in the Levant, see Brian Boyd 2007.

47. As William Boyd and Michael Watts (1997) remind us, though, industrial animal production originates not with pigs but with chickens. For yet another discussion on the political economy of pork production, see B. Weiss 2012.

48. The "terminal" quality of the pig is especially evident in the fact that many people with whom I have spoken—at 4H gatherings, county fairs, swine research centers, and university-based farms—often could not tell me how long a pig could live because all animals they had encountered, even over the course of decades of experience, had ended up either in laboratories or at the slaughterhouse within the first two years of life. As one husbandry specialist with forty years experience with pigs told me in 2008, "what we know about their longevity springs from anecdotal accounts about pet pigs—I've never seen an old pig die." For such an account, see Montgomery 2006.

49. Among the more astonishing innovations, at least from a lay perspective, to be displayed in the past decade occurred during a conference in Australia involving one lab's successful attempts to produce pigs within the same litter that would glow different colors under ultraviolet light so that their genetic differences could be detected with ease without the use of invasive procedures.

50. For a wonderful critique of the quantification of proximity, see Marks 2003.

51. Such errors are extremely rare. If left untreated (again, highly unusual), the more severe and potentially life-threatening responses include fever, chills, hypotension, hemorrhaging, anaphylactic shock, and a form of pulmonary distress known as transfusion-associated acute lung injury (or TRALI).

CHAPTER THREE. ARTIFICIAL LIFE
This chapter is dedicated with love to Uncle Wally (Wallace) Kreisman, who died in 2012. Our conversations over the years inspired the analysis presented here.

1. Project Bionics is a web-based archive sponsored jointly by the American Society for Artificial Internal Organs (ASAIO) and the Smithsonian Museum (see http://echo.gmu.edu/bionics, accessed June 2012; see also Littleton 2004).

2. Consider, for instance, Herman Broers's (2007) passing reference to "the 'heart boys'" (172) of the University of Utah in his biography of Willem Kolff. Until very recently, women involved in bioengineering generally worked as lab and office assistants. Sometimes they were researchers' wives. They appear intermittently in lab photos but generally remain unidentified.

3. For simplicity's sake, I employ the term "bioengineer" as shorthand for "biomechanical engineer" and, further, I apply it to all professionals who work directly on artificial organ design, whether or not they hold degrees in engineering. All specialists interviewed for this chapter are members of (or at least attend the annual meetings of) a venerated international association that both specializes in bioengineering and claims to be among the oldest transplant associations in the world. In those cases where an individual's training in another field is relevant (such as veterinary science or clinical medicine), I make note of this in the text.

4. I broach this topic in chapter 4.

5. "LVAS," or "left ventricular assist system," is a corporate embellishment of the more standard "LVAD," or "left ventricular assist device."

6. According to biographer David Friedman (2007, 9–11), Carrel was a target of anti-vivisectionists, who sought ultimately to restrict his research through legislative measures. Carrel's success in 1908 in saving the life of the five-day-old daughter of Adrian V. S. Lambert, a Columbia medical school professor, helped defeat the bill, using the argument that animal research had informed his life-saving surgical techniques.

7. David Friedman (2007, 5) describes Carrel as "nearly a foot shorter" than Lindbergh. This was Carrel's second appearance on *Time*'s cover. As noted in chapter 2, the first was Sept. 16, 1935.

8. Carrel is credited with developing the first antiseptic (sodium hypochlorite, buffered with sodium bicarbonate) while serving as a surgeon in the French

army in World War I (D. Friedman 2007, 2). Within his lab at the Rockefeller Institute in New York, Carrel initiated a range of surgical innovations, many of which revolutionized sterile surgical practices. Hand and face washing, for instance, were essential. A special obsession was his insistence that surgery be conducted in a room where the walls, ceiling, and floor were painted black, and with a skylight above. Staff dressed in what might best be called "surgical blacks," including a hood of sorts that exposed only the eyes. Carrel distinguished himself from others within the operating theater by being the only one to wear a white cap. According to Carrel, these practices not only helped to prevent visual distraction but also enabled the surgeon to detect the presence of potentially infectious agents (e.g., dust and other particles) because they could be spotted with ease against the dark background (D. Friedman 2007, 14–16). This is likewise described in the *Time* article that accompanied the cover image (Men in Black 1938).

9. Lindbergh did so with the indispensable assistance of the staff glassblower, Otto Hopf (D. Friedman 2007, 33).

10. As Joshua Lederberg, former president of what became known as Rockefeller University, recounted to me in Jan. 2008, he himself achieved this honor at the even more "precocious age of 33" in 1958. To view *Time*'s cover on June 13, 1938, showing Carrel and Lindbergh with a perfusion pump, go to http://www.time.com/time/covers/0,16641,19380613,00.html (accesses June 1, 2013).

11. Key components of the perfusion pump included the ability to supply an appropriate gas mixture to the chamber to oxygenate excised tissue, a culture broth that could serve as a sterile environment, and proper nutrients delivered in pulses that approximated the functions of the heart (see D. Friedman 2007, 62–74). A *Time* reporter offered the following lively, detailed description, where the ultimate goal was to maintain an organ outside the body so that perhaps it could heal and then be reimplanted in a patient: "Looking like a twist of vitrified bowel oozing out of a clear glass bottle, the Lindbergh perfusion pump consists of three chambers one above the other. The organ to be studied lies on the slanting glass floor of the topmost. Nutritious fluid from the lowest or reservoir chamber is driven up a glass tube connected with the organ's artery, to and through the organ by pulsating gas pressure. After passing through the organ, the fluid runs down into the central or pressure equalization chamber, back to the reservoir chamber. There are no moving parts. The whole apparatus is actuated by compressed air from a tank, controlled by a rotary valve which creates the pulsating pressure. Nonabsorbent cotton in bulbs through which the gases pass, keeps germs from getting into the apparatus, the organ, or the fluid. Thus the 'heart' action of the pump. To imitate lungs, there is an inlet for air or other gas into the blood. To remove the waste products of this disembodied living [*sic*].

Dr. Carrel needs a glass 'kidney.' Colonel Lindbergh, 3,000 miles away from the Rockefeller Institute, this week is cogitating that problem. In this perfusion pump Dr. Carrel has kept thyroid glands, ovaries, hearts, kidneys and pancreases of guinea pigs and cats alive for as long as 30 days. He has caused pancreases to produce insulin; thyroids, thyroid hormone" (Men in Black 1938).

12. Lindbergh was not the first aviation engineer to enter Carrel's laboratory to assist him in his longstanding determination to develop an aseptic perfusion device. As reported in *Time* (Men in Black 1938), "By 1929 Dr. Carrel had reached the point at which his work was being seriously retarded for lack of a germ-proof pump. A German flier and aeronautical engineer, Heinz Rosenberger, whom he had imported from Berlin, built a self-contained pump with a piston oscillated from outside by electromagnets. This 'failed completely.' Rosenberger eventually retired to Sandy Hook, Conn., to make moving pictures of microorganisms," on which he subsequently collaborated with Carrel.

13. David Friedman (2007, 45–48) offers an extensive account of this partnership in his work *The Immortalists*, which serves as an invaluable source for my discussion here. He argues that, for Lindbergh, the quest to extend human life evolved later to include a conviction driven by nationalistic and racialized eugenics.

14. From 1935 to 1939, nearly 900 perfusion experiments occurred in Carrel's lab. Although it fell into disuse when Carrel was forced into retirement at age 65 in 1939, the apparatus (which had become known as the Lindbergh RIMR, for Rockefeller Institute for Medical Research) was revived in 1964 at the U.S. Naval Medical Research Institute with Lindbergh present (Dutkowski et al. 2008).

15. High concentrations of urea and salt were filtered from the patient's blood by passing the latter through a water bath and porous container. The principle at work was that high concentrations of these substances would move to areas of less concentration where possible (see Brown 2009).

16. More specifically, as reported by Eli Friedman (2009), Kolff initiated postgraduate work at the University of Groningen under the direction of Leo Polak Daniels, who was Jewish. Following Germany's invasion of the Netherlands in 1940, Polak Daniels and his wife committed suicide and Kolff resigned, "unwilling to work for his Nazi-appointed successor" (180).

17. The boy survived and later became a dentist based in the Netherlands (Brown 2009; E. Friedman 2009).

18. As is common in bioengineering, several researchers were simultaneously at work designing artificial kidneys alongside Kolff's efforts. A year after Kolff's breakthrough, Nils Alwall in Sweden published findings on his own work in 1947, followed by Gordon Murray in Toronto in 1948. Kolff had built four artificial kidneys, which he hid in 1944 during the war; he subsequently donated

these to hospitals in London, Poland, Canada, and the United States (the last, more specifically, to the Jewish Mount Sinai Hospital in New York) (Broers 2007, 112–13).

19. According to Broers (2007, 156–57), who interviewed Kolff's colleague Yukihiko Nosé (who would himself make significant strides in artificial heart design), institutional jealousies led Kolff to search for posts that would enable him to leave Cleveland. One possibility was Baylor University in Houston, yet Michael DeBakey's presence as a "great competitor in the race to make the first artificial heart" precluded this. Kolff was encouraged to move to Salt Lake City and join an expanding program under the now-legendary transplant surgeon Keith Reemtsma, well known at the time for his attempts at xenotransplants in New Orleans; Kolff's responsibilities in Utah entailed establishing a new program in artificial organ design. (For more on Kolff, see also Sharp 2011c.)

20. See http://healthcare.utah.edu/publicaffairs/spotlight/KolffMemoriam.html, accessed June 15, 2012.

21. Kantrowitz is widely celebrated in transplant medicine as the first to have performed a pediatric heart transplant, which he did only three days after Christiaan Barnard's historic attempt in South Africa involving an adult patient. Kantrowitz is thus also credited with performing the first heart transplant in the United States. For a discussion of the rivalries involved here, see Starzl 1992.

22. Olsen is a veterinary surgeon who worked with Kolff at the University of Utah in the 1970s and 1980s. He is widely considered a leader in the field, and his corpus of experiments with calves defines an important step in the development of implantable heart technology.

23. For a photo of Kolff and Clifford Kwan-Gett posing with their prototype of an artificial heart in 1968, see Broers 2007, 161. This and other photos provide an important archive today because all of Kolff's lab's artificial heart models dating back to 1957 were lost in a fire in 1973, presumably caused by a lab assistant who had committed fraud. Only the "Jarvik" heart was retrieved from the smoldering remains by its eponymous researcher (Broers 2007, 170–71).

24. The cumbersome external drive system was originally modeled after a milking machine used on dairy farms. According to Broers (2007), on a much earlier occasion Kolff's Cleveland team designed a "Maytag washing machine-kidney" as a possible prototype for home-based dialysis. Says Broers, "Washing-machine manufacturer Maytag was less than charmed with Kolff's idea" (152; see also photo on 152).

25. Other celebrated figures include Adrian Kantrowitz, who in 1966 at Maimonides Medical Center in Brooklyn, N.Y., implanted the first partial mechanical heart device (now known as an LVAD) in a patient. Domingo Liotta—a pioneer in artificial heart research who had worked with animals in France and

Argentina—joined Michael DeBakey in early LVAD work at Methodist Hospital in Houston in 1966; later, he worked with Denton Cooley (DeBakey's former-colleague-turned-rival) on bridge-to-transplant research involving yet another mechanical heart device in 1969 at the Texas Heart Institute in Houston. The celebrated surgeon William DeVries worked alongside Kolff with Barney Clark in Utah in 1982. Expertise on mechanical hearts extends well beyond the field of medicine and includes such expert inventors with medical training as Robert Jarvik, after whom several devices are named, and Donald Olsen, a veterinarian whose animal experiments had a significant effect on surgical outcomes. This is hardly an exhaustive list, but it does highlight major strides in artificial heart design over the course of the first thirty years of activity (http://en.wikipedia.org/wiki/Artificial_heart, accessed June 5, 2012; assorted interviews with me; fieldnotes).

26. Carrel also worked to transform the delivery of medical care in France during World War II (Malinin 1979). War often throws together men of very different backgrounds, a process that may well facilitate "tinkering" with new ideas or technologies. I thank Janelle Taylor for this insight.

27. See, for instance, http://en.wikipedia.org/wiki/Artificial_heart, accessed June 13, 2012; Lavietes 2003; and Ohse 1993. Photographs of Sewell's erector-set device can be viewed on the web page of the Eli Whitney Museum and Workshop of Yale University, http://www.eliwhitney.org/new/museum/-gilbert-project/-man/a-c-gilbert-scientific-toymaker-essays-arts-and-sci-ences-october-3, accessed June 19, 2012.

28. Thus, the inventive bioengineer provides a wonderful amalgamation of Lévi-Strauss's (1966) comparative categories of the *bricoleur* and the engineer.

29. I must stress, however, that bioengineering's premier professional organization has pushed hard in recent years to "youthanize" (as one member jokingly put it) its ranks, most evident in the establishment of a special division for its junior members. I have attended annual meetings spread over a decade and have witnessed significant shifts not only in membership but also in leadership.

30. The heart is composed in large part of four chambers: the upper right and left atria, and the lower right and left ventricles. The left ventricle is most often associated with heart failure because it is the chamber that receives oxygenated blood from the lungs that then needs to be pushed up through the aorta and on throughout the body. It is more muscular, and characterized by greater pressure, than the right ventricle, which receives deoxygenated blood that is then fed back a short distance into the lungs. Some patients do indeed require RVADs (right ventricular assist devices) or, in some cases, double VAD assistance when both ventricles are weak and/or damaged.

31. I frequently attend trade shows where a range of devices intended to replace body parts are marketed, and I had only recently encountered a "display" by one of Legstrom's competitors where the "prototype" was a live woman who sported two high-tech prosthetic legs. Because of the requirements of the prostheses' design parameters, her standing height was around 6'2".

32. This reference to Zeno's Paradox pokes fun both at those who employ the scientific method and at engineers.

33. During a more informal interaction with two other female engineers, we were speaking of how academic departments in this field are overwhelmingly male. At one point in the conversation, one of the two women stood up and, with a grabbing gesture, tugged forcefully up on an imaginary pair of very large testicles in front of her groin area, coupled with a few pelvic thrusts, and then, as she sat back down, her friend, laughing, said, "It's, true, to make it you gotta be like the Big Boys."

34. I drifted into the art department, where I learned I could do all the same work (by using many of the same tools) in miniature.

35. Faulkner (2000) describes in other quarters the respect expressed for women's "softer" skills and qualities. As testimonies from Blalock and several other female bioengineers of her generation demonstrate, though, their experiences lack the benign qualities Faulkner describes.

36. I thank my colleague Mary Gordon for this idea: she once described herself to me as "very dog dependent."

37. When I worked within a lab complex in Cambridge, Mass., in the early 1980s, one of the duties assigned to postdoctoral students was to drive around town at night looking for stray dogs who could then be put to use in heart research experiments.

38. My sense is that the sex of the animal may matter here, too: calves are generally young bulls, whereas sheep are ewes. I have had very little contact with anyone who has worked with goats. There may be something at work here in terms of how researchers—who are overwhelmingly male—relate to young bulls, although this is a mere hunch based on anecdotal data. Note that the female calf Diana (discussed in the text below) was sacrificed to save her male sibling, Charles. The names they share with the royal British couple are a coincidence (their human counterparts met in 1980).

39. This statement also has special bearing on the humane management of an animal. That is, an animal that suffers compromises research outcomes.

40. When shown these photos, Mette Svendsen, who writes on the use of laboratory pigs (Svendsen and Koch forthcoming), remarked that they were eerily reminiscent of family photos.

41. For a photo of young Olsen with Phred, a sheep implanted with a heart device, see http://www.deseretnews.com/article/695230569/82-heart-implant-sparked-progress.html?pg = all (from the University of Utah),accessed Sept. 22, 2012.

42. See http://www.syncardia.com/component/option,com_arttimeline/ Itemid,707/timelineid,1, accessed June 13, 2012, and http://en.wikipedia.org/ wiki/Artificial_heart, accessed June 16, 2012.

43. The ad then points readers to www.jarvikheart.com. It appeared in the program for the annual ASAIO conference, June 2005, Washington, D.C.

44. To disguise Houghton's identity would do disservice to an extraordinary individual, and thus I employ his real name here in my very brief overview of his remarkable life (1938–2007). Any omissions or errors are mine alone. For an archived radio broadcast on Houghton's life, see the BBC Radio 4's obituaries program "Last Word," http://www.bbc.co.uk/radio4/news/lastword_04jan2008. shtml, aired Jan. 4, 2008, accessed July 6, 2012.

45. Houghton has also written on his life as a devout Catholic, and he assisted James Hughes (2004) on a work addressing the ethics of bionic implants (see Garreau 2007).

46. The life history is an important methodological component of ethnographic field research, and thus I have assembled many such histories over the course of more than two decades working as an anthropologist. Space restrictions prevent me from detailing Houghton's full biography here, but it is among the most memorable life accounts I have ever had the privilege of hearing. Long before he received a surgically implanted LVAD, Houghton had worked as an English teacher at a Dominican mission in Mozambique; he was widowed with an infant son to care for; he trained as a psychotherapist back home in the United Kingdom, then ran a hostel for disturbed teens and, subsequently, a "settlement house" for impoverished women; he founded a debt counseling service and co-founded the National Association for the Childless with his second wife, with whom he was a key figure in offering early testimony regarding in-vitro fertilization; he worked as an AIDs and palliative care counselor as early as the late 1980s; and he served as a foster parent for numerous children and, in at least one case, a victim of torture (interview June 11, 2005).

47. Their surgeon, William DeVries, was born in the Netherlands in 1943 and was trained in medicine at the University of Utah, working with Kolff's team in the 1980s. Clark and Schroeder were implanted with a cumbersome device known as the Jarvik-7, named after inventor Robert Jarvik. (Schroeder was able to travel using a fifteen-pound portable driver system.) Three other patients—two in Louisville, one in Sweden—frequently go unreferenced (see http://www. jarvikheart.com/basic.asp?id = 69, accessed July 7, 2012).

48. See http://www.thetransplantlog.com under "Sound" entry, accessed July 7, 2012; see also Wainwright and Wynne 2008.

49. I have been unable to confirm whether or not this was true.

CHAPTER FOUR. TEMPORALITY AND SOCIAL DESIRE IN ANTICIPATORY SCIENCE

1. As Mol and her colleagues (2010) demonstrate, "tinkering" may also be conceived as a form of "care." I thank Janelle Taylor for alerting me to this possibility.

2. The revived presence of pharmaceutical and technical firms at MIT and other campuses across the United States blurs only further this distinction between academic and industrial science.

3. These strategies are reminiscent of what Glenn Davis Stone (forthcoming) identifies as a form of "effective ignorance" or "agnotology" (or "ignorance creating" strategies)—albeit, in the context of bioengineering conferences, data are deliberately withheld (as opposed to avoidance of certain research topics, as Stone describes). Nevertheless, he offers an intriguing framework on why certain knowledge remains unknown in domains of science. His work alerts us to moments within experimental transplant science when the political dangers associated with melding academic science and industry surface, or where the dangers of the technology itself remain unknown through deliberate efforts to block knowledge or, as Stone shows, new research. Although beyond the purview of this book, this is, I believe, most certainly the case where patients' experiences are concerned. Within transplant medicine, for instance, involved clinicians were long reticent to track patient survival beyond three or even five years, fearful they might find few who were still alive. Similarly, two decades ago I struggled to find anyone willing to discuss, much less study, the effects of massive doses of immunosuppressive steroids on child growth (see Sharp 2006b).

4. DARPA is well known among engineers as a source of funding and prize money for inventions that could have military applications. Among its most celebrated events is the longstanding Grand Challenge for driverless vehicles, an event especially popular among robotics experts.

5. See, for instance, http://www.govtrack.us/congress/bills/111/s1435, accessed Sept. 11, 2012. Although the bill had failed in 2009, a version did in fact pass in Brownback's home state, and attempts were revived yet again at the national level in September 2012.

6. Interestingly, among a well-informed, news-savvy public, such measures are perceived as absurdist and comical: on a recent airing of "Wait Wait . . . Don't Tell Me!," host Peter Sagal and the week's panelists made a string of jokes about the impossibility of creating human-animal hybrids and how Senator Sam

Brownback's most recently proposed bill was therefore a waste of time (NPR 2012; see also Chillig 2010).

7. The term "translational science" currently proliferates in many other fields, too. The concept itself is not, however, that new. Over half a century ago, Thomas Kuhn spoke of the importance of scientists engaging in "translation for the layman" (Kuhn 1962, 20, as noted in Coen 2013, 11).

8. I have encountered this expansion of the meaning of "translational" in other contexts as well. Bioethicists, for instance, speak of their own work as "translational" because they "translate" the meanings and relevance of morality among clinicians, researchers, and the public. Others evoke "translation" in reference to the marketing of discoveries: e.g., one transforms the abstractness of an idea, device, or technique into something that can be made practical to clinicians and other "end users."

9. At the very moment when Kenyon made this point, another senior Canadian researcher stopped by to say hello, and she let him know "We're talking right now about vertical and horizontal integration."

10. Such an approach is highly reminiscent of the biotech neighborhoods that have cropped up in recent years in Singapore (a site where several xeno experts have relocated their labs because the scientific freedoms they experience there surpass experiences in the United States, the United Kingdom, and Australia). As described to me by contributors who participated in a conference on Asian biotech (see Ong and Chen 2010), planned neighborhoods include housing intermixed with research laboratories and, furthermore, a quite literal element of "transparency" when laboratories have large windows opening out onto public streets.

CONCLUSION

1. I am indebted to Janelle Taylor, who urged me to consider this theme more carefully.

Abadie, Roberto. 2010. *The Professional Guinea Pig: Big Pharma and the Risky World of Human Subjects*. Durham: Duke University Press.

ABC (Australian Broadcasting Corporation). 1997. Animal Transplants. *Four Corners* (with Murray McLaughlin), aired Aug. 25. Sydney: ABC.

Allan, Jonathan S. 1996. Xenotransplantation at a Crossroads: Prevention Versus Progress. *Nature Medicine* 2 (1): 18–21.

Altman, Lawrence K. 1983. Barney Clark Dies in 112th Day with Permanent Artificial Heart. *New York Times*, Mar. 24.

———. 1986. William Schroeder Dies 620 Days After Receiving Artificial Heart. *New York Times*, Aug. 8.

———. 2000. Keith Reemtsma, 74, Pioneer in Medical Transplants, Dies (obituary). *New York Times*, Feb. 10.

Archer, Kirstie, and Faith McLellan. 2002. Controversy Surrounds Proposed Xenotransplant Trial. *The Lancet* 359: 949.

Atala, Anthony. 2005. Tissue Engineered Artificial Organs: Current Concepts and Changing Trends. Keynote Lecture, 51st Annual Conference of the American Society for Artifician Organs (ASAIO), Washington, D.C.

Auchincloss Jr., Hugh. 1988. Xenogeneic Transplantation: A Review. *Transplantation* 46 (1): 1–20.

Bach, Fritz H. 1996. Transplanting Porcine Hearts to Humans: Understanding the Mechanisms Gives Cause for Optimism. *BMJ* 312: 651–52.

Bach, Fritz H., J. A. Fishman, N. Daniels, J. Proimos, B. Anderson, C. B. Carpenter, L. Forrow, S. C. Robson, and H. V. Fineberg. 1998. Uncertainty in Xenotransplantation: Individual Benefits Versus Collective Risk. *Nature Medicine* 4 (2): 141–44.

Bach, Fritz H., and Adrian J. Ivinson. 2002. A Shrewd and Ethical Approach to Xenotransplantation. *Trends in Biotechnology* 20 (3): 129–31.

Bach, Fritz H., Adrian J. Ivinson, and H. E. Judge Christopher Weeramantry. 2001. Ethical and Legal Issues in Technology: Xenotransplantation. *American Journal of Law and Medicine* 27: 283–300.

Banner, Michael. 1999. *Christian Ethics and Contemporary Moral Problems*. Cambridge: Cambridge University Press.

———. Forthcoming. What Is Morality? Moral Philosophy, Social Anthropology and the Ethics of Everyday Life. Unpublished manuscript.

Bateson, Gregory. 1958. *Naven: A Survey of the Problems Suggested by a Composite Picture of the Culture of a New Guinea Tribe Drawn from Three Points of View*. Stanford: Stanford University Press.

BBC (British Broadcasting Corporation). 1999. The History of Xenotransplantation. BBC News, Sci/Tech section, http://news.bbc.co.uk/2/hi/science/nature/425120.stm (accessed Aug. 19).

Beauchamp, Tom L., and James F. Childress. 1979. *Principles of Biomedical Ethics*. Oxford: Oxford University Press.

Beidelman, Thomas O. 1993. *Moral Imagination in Kaguru Modes of Thought*. Washington, D.C.: Smithsonian Institution Press.

Bellah, Robert. 1979. The Quest for the Self: Individualism, Morality, Politics. In *Interpretative Social Science*, edited by P. Rabinow and W. M. Sullivan, 365–83. Berkeley: University of California Press.

Benedict, Ruth. 1934. Anthropology and the Abnormal. *Journal of General Psychology* 10 (1): 59–80.

Biles, Jeremy. 2007. *Ecce Monstrum: Georges Bataille and the Sacrifice of Form*. New York: Fordham University Press.

Bille, Mikkel, Frida Hastrup, and Tim Flohr, eds. 2010. *An Anthropology of Absence: Materialisations of Transcendence and Loss*. Copenhagen: Springer Press.

Birmingham, Karen. 1999. WHO Hosts Web Discussion on Xenotransplantation Policy. *Nature Medicine* 5 (6): 595.

Bloch, Maurice. 1995. People into Places. In *The Anthropology of Landscape: Perspectives on Place and Space*, edited by E. Hirsch and M. O'Hanlon, 63–77. Oxford: Clarendon Press.

Blum, Deborah. 1994. *The Monkey Wars*. New York: Oxford University Press.

Bock, Gregory, and Jamie Goode, eds. 2007. *Tinkering: The Microevolution of Development (from the Symposium on Tinkering, Novartis Foundation, London, July 11–13, 2006)*. Chichester, U.K.: John Wiley & Sons.

Bourdieu, Pierre. 1994. Structures, Habitus, Power: Basis for a Theory of Symbolic Power (1977). In *Culture/Power/History: A Reader in Contemporary Social Theory*, edited by N. Dirks, G. Eley, and S. Ortner, 155–99. Princeton: Princeton University Press.

Boyd, Brian. 2007. *People and Animals in Levantine Prehistory: 20,000–8,000 BC*. Cambridge: Cambridge University Press.

Boyd, William, and Michael J. Watts. 1997. Agro-Industrial Just-in-Time: The Chicken Industry and Postwar American Capitalism. In *Globalising Food: Agrarian Questions and Global Restructuring*, edited by D. Goodman and M. J. Watts, 139–66. New York: Routledge.

Brodwin, Paul, ed. 2000. *Biotechnology and Culture: Bodies, Anxieties, Ethics*. Bloomington: Indiana University Press.

———. 2013. *Everyday Ethics: Voices from the Front Line of Community Psychiatry*. Berkeley: University of California Press.

Broers, Herman. 2007. *Inventor for Life: The Story of W. J. Kolff, Father of Artificial Organs*. Translated by K. Ashton. Kampen, the Netherlands: B&V Media Publishers.

Brown, David. 2009. Willem J. Kolff, 97: Doctor Invented Kidney Dialysis Machine, Artificial Organs (obituary). *Washington Post*, Feb. 13.

Calne, Roy. 2005. Xenografting—The Future of Transplantation, and Always Will Be? *Xenotransplantation* 12 (1): 5–6.

Caplan, A. L. 1992. Is Xenografting Morally Wrong? *Transplantation Proceedings* 24 (2): 722–27.

Carrel, Alexis. 1935. *Man, The Unknown (L'Homme, cet inconnu)*. New York: Harper and Brothers.

Chillag, Ian. 2010. The New Animal Hybrids. In *Wait Wait . . . Don't Blog Me!* National Public Radio, Sept. 14, 2012. http://www.npr.org/blogs/waitwait/2010/09/14/129859451/the-new-animal-hybrids.

Clark, Margaret A. 1993. Medical Anthropology and the Redefining of Human Nature. *Human Organization* 52 (3): 233–42.

———. 1999. This Little Piggy Went to Market: The Xenotransplantation and Xenozoonose Debate. *Journal of Law, Medicine and Ethics* 27: 137–52.

Coen, Deborah R. 2013. *The Earthquake Observers: Disaster Science from Lisbon to Richter*. Chicago: Chicago University Press.

Cook, Peta S. 2006. Science Stories: Selecting the Source Animal for Xenotransplantation. In *Social Change in the 21st Century*, edited by C. Hopkinson and C. Hall. Conference Proceedings, Centre for Social Change Research, Queensland University of Technology, Brisbane, Australia.

Cooper, David K. C. 2007. René Kuss's Clinical Experience with Pig Kidney Transplantation in 1966 (letter to the editors). *Xenotransplantation* 14: 93.

Cooper, David K. C., Bernd Gollackner, and David H. Sachs. 2002. Will the Pig Solve the Transplantation Backlog? *Annual Review of Medicine* 53: 133–47.

Cooper, David K. C., A. M. Keogh, J. Brink, P. A. Corris, W. Klepetko, R. N. Pierson, M. Schmoeckel, R. Shirakura, and L. Warner Stevenson. 2000. Report of the Xenotransplantation Advisory Committee of the International Society for Heart and Lung Transplantation: The Present Status of Xenotransplantation and Its Potential Role in the Treatment of End-Stage Cardiac and Pulmonary Diseases. *Journal of Heart and Lung Transplantation* 19: 1125–65.

Cooper, David K. C., and Robert Paul Lanza. 2000. *Xeno: The Promise of Transplanting Animal Organs into Humans*. Oxford: Oxford University Press.

Copeman, Jacob. 2005. Veinglory: Exploring Processes of Blood Transfer Between Persons. *Journal of the Royal Anthropological Institute* 11: 465–85.

Dahl, Roald. 1964. *Charlie and the Chocolate Factory*. London: Alfred A. Knopf.

Das, Veena. 2012. Ordinary Ethics. In *A Companion to Moral Anthropology*, edited by D. Fassin, 133–49. Hoboken, N.J.: John Wiley & Sons.

DelVecchio Good, Mary-Jo. 2001. The Biotechnical Embrace. *Culture, Medicine and Psychiatry* 25 (4): 395–410.

———. 2007. The Biotechnical Embrace and the Medical Imaginary. In *Subjectivity: Ethnographic Investigations*, edited by J. Biehl, B. Good, and A. Kleinman, 362–80. Berkeley: University of California Press.

DelVecchio Good, Mary-Jo, Byron J. Good, Cynthia Schaffer, and Stuart E. Lind. 1990. American Oncology and the Discourse on Hope. *Culture, Medicine and Psychiatry* 14: 59–79.

DelVecchio Good, Mary-Jo, with Esther Mwaikambo, Erastus Amayo, and James M'Imunya Machoki. 1999. Clinical Realities and Moral Dilemmas: Contrasting Perspectives from Academic Medicine in Kenya, Tanzania, and America. *Daedalus* 128 (4): 167–96.

Deschamps, Jack-Yves, Françoise A. Roux, Pierre Saï, and Edouard Gouin. 2005. History of Xenotransplantation. *Xenotransplantation* 12 (2): 91–109.

Descola, Philippe, and Gísli Pálsson. 1996. Introduction. In *Nature and Society: Anthropological Perspectives*, edited by P. Descola and G. Pálsson, 1–21. London: Routledge.

De Witte, Joke I., and Henk Ten Have. 1997. Ownership of Genetic Material and Information. *Social Science and Medicine* 45 (1): 51–60.

DOH-UK (Department of Health-UK). 1997. *A Report by the Advisory Group on the Ethics of Xenotransplantation [The Kennedy Report]*. London: DOH-UK.

Donnelley, Strachan. 1999. The Moral Landscape of Xenotransplantation [or: Casting Pearls Before Miniature, Transgenic Swine]. Manuscript, Humans and Nature Program, Cold Spring Harbor, N.Y., 3 pp.

Douglas, Mary. 1966. *Purity and Danger: An Analysis of Concepts of Pollution and Taboo*. New York: Praeger.

Durkheim, Emile. (1897) 1997. *Suicide: A Study in Sociology*. Translated by J. A. Spaulding and G. Simpson. New York: The Free Press.

Dutkowski, P., O. de Rougemont, and P.-A. Clavien. 2008. Alexis Carrel: Genius, Innovator, and Ideologist. *American Journal of Transplantation* 8: 1998–2003.

Edel, May M., and Abraham Edel. 1959. *Anthropology and Ethics*. Springfield, Ill.: Thomas.

Evans-Prichard, E. E. 1937. *Witchcraft, Oracles and Magic among the Azande*. Oxford: Oxford University Press.

Fassin, Didier, ed. 2012. *A Companion to Moral Anthropology*. Hoboken, N.J.: John Wiley & Sons.

Faubion, James D. 2011. *An Anthropology of Ethics*. Cambridge: Cambridge University Press.

Faulkner, Alex, and Julie Kent. 2001. Innovation and Regulation in Human Implant Technologies: Developing Comparative Approaches. *Social Science and Medicine* 53: 895–913.

Faulkner, Wendy. 2000. Dualisms, Hierarchies and Gender in Engineering. *Social Studies of Science* 30 (5): 759–92.

Ferry, Elizabeth Emma, and Mandana E. Limbert, eds. 2008. *Timely Assets: The Politics of Resources and Their Temporalities*. Santa Fe: School for Advanced Research Press.

Fischer, Michael M. J. 2001. Ethnographic Critique and Technoscientific Narratives: The Old Mole, Ethical Plateaux, and the Governance of Emergent Biosocial Polities. *Culture, Medicine, and Psychiatry* 25: 355–93.

Fitzpatrick, Laura. 2009. A Brief History of Heart Transplants. *Time*, Nov. 16. http://www.time.com/time/health/article/0,8599,1939493,00.html (accessed Mar. 1, 2010).

Foucault, Michel. 1984. On the Genealogy of Ethics: An Overview of Work in Progress. In *The Foucault Reader*, edited by P. Rabinow, 340–72. New York: Pantheon.

Fox, Renée C. 1959. *Experiment Perilous*. Glencoe, Ill.: The Free Press.

———. 1996. Afterthoughts: Continuing Reflections on Organ Transplantation. In *Organ Transplantation: Meanings and Realities*, edited by S. J. Youngner, R. C. Fox, and L. J. O'Connell, 252–72. Madison: University of Wisconsin Press.

Fox, Renée C., and Judith P. Swazey. 1978. *The Courage to Fail: A Social View of Organ Transplants and Dialysis*. Chicago: University of Chicago Press.

———. 1992. *Spare Parts: Organ Replacement in American Society*. Oxford: Oxford University Press.

———. 2004. "He Knows that Machine Is His Mortality": Old and New Social and Cultural Patterns in the Clinical Trial of the AbioCor Artificial Heart. *Perspectives in Biology and Medicine* 47 (1): 74–99.

Franklin, Sarah. 1997. *Embodied Progress: A Cultural Account of Assisted Conception*. New York: Routledge.

———. 2003. Kinship, Genes and Cloning: Life After Dolly. In *Genetic Nature/Culture: Anthropology and Science Beyond the Two-Culture Divide*, edited by A. H. Goodman, D. Heath, and M. S. Lindee, 95–110. Berkeley: University of California Press.

———. 2007. *Dolly Mixtures: The Remaking of Genealogy*. Durham: Duke University Press.

Franklin, Sarah, and Margaret Lock. 2003. Animation and Cessation: The Remaking of Life and Death. In *Remaking Life and Death: Toward an Anthropology of the Biosciences*. S. Franklin and M. Lock, eds. Pp. 3–22. Santa Fe: School of American Research Press.

Friedman, David M. 2007. *The Immortalists: Charles Lindbergh, Dr. Alexis Carrel, and Their Daring Quest to Live Forever*. New York: Harper Perennial.

Friedman, Eli A. 2009. Willem Johan "Pim" Kolff: Bionics for Humans in Any Season, Feb. 14, 1911–Feb. 11, 2009. *Dialysis and Transplantation* 38 (5): 180–82.

Fuentes, Agustin. 2007. Monkey and Human Interconnections: The Wild, the Captive, and the In-between. In *Where the Wild Things Are Now: Domestication Reconsidered*, edited by R. Cassidy and M. Mullin, 123–45. New York: Berg.

Garreau, Joel. 2007. His Heart Whirs Anew. *Washington Post*, Aug. 11.

Gibson, William. 1984. *Neuromancer*. New York: Ace Books.

Gil, Gideon. 1989. The Artificial Heart Juggernaut. *The Hastings Center Report* 19 (2): 24–31.

Gluckman, Max. 1963. The Magic of Despair. In his *Order and Rebellion in Tribal Africa*, 135–45. Glencoe: The Free Press.

Gorman, James. 2011a. Chimps' Days in Labs May Be Dwindling. *New York Times*, Nov. 15, pp. D1, D4.

———. 2011b. Elevation of the Chimp May Reshape Research. *New York Times*, Dec. 20, pp. D1, D6.

———. 2011c. U.S. Will Not Finance New Research Involving Chimps. *New York Times*, Dec. 16, p. A26.

Gorovitz, Samuel. 1987. The Artificial Heart: Questions to Ask, and Not to Ask. In *Human Organ Transplantation: Societal, Medical-Legal, Regulatory, and Reimbursement Issues*, edited by D. H. Cowan, J. A. Kantorowitz, J. Moskowitz, and P. H. Rheinstein, 380–85. Ann Arbor, Mich.: Health Administration Press in Cooperation with the American Society of Law and Medicine.

Gray, Chris Hables. 2001. *Cyborg Citizen: Politics in the Postmodern Age*. New York: Routledge.

Groth, Carl G. 2008. Looking Back, Heading Forward. *Xenotransplantation* 15: 1–2.

Guyer, Jane I. 2007. Prophecy and the Near Future: Thoughts on Macroeconomic, Evangelical, and Punctuated Time. *American Ethnologist* 34 (3): 409–21.

Hamilton, Anita. 2001. Inventions of the Year / Your Health / Abiocor Artificial Heart. *Time*, Nov. 19.

Haraway, Donna J. 1991. *Simians, Cyborgs, and Women: The Reinvention of Nature.* New York: Routledge.

———. 1992. The Promises of Monsters: A Regenerative Politics for Inappropriate/d Others. In *Cultural Studies*, edited by L. Grossberg, C. Nelson, and P. Treichler, 295–337. New York: Routledge.

———. 1997. *Modest_Witness@Second_Millennium.FemaleMan^c_Meets_ OncoMouse^TM: Feminism and Technoscience.* New York: Routledge.

———. 2003. *The Companion Species Manifesto: Dogs, People, and Significant Otherness.* Chicago: Prickly Paradigm Press.

Heintz, Monica, ed. 2009. *The Anthropology of Moralities.* New York: Berghahn Books.

Helmreich, Stefan. 2009. *Alien Ocean: Anthropological Voyages in Microbial Seas.* Berkeley: University of California Press.

Hogle, Linda F. 1995. Tales from the Cryptic: Technology Meets Organism in the Living Cadaver. In *The Cyborg Handbook*, edited by C. H. Gray, 203–16. New York: Routledge.

Houghton, Peter. 2001. *On Death and Not Dying.* London: Jessica Kingsley Publishers.

Howell, Signe, ed. 1997. *The Ethnography of Moralities.* London: Routledge.

Hughes, James. 2004. *Citizen Cyborg: Why Democratic Societies Must Respond to the Redesigned Human of the Future.* Cambridge, Mass.: Westview Press.

Ingold, Tim. 1980. *Hunters, Pastoralists and Ranchers: Reindeer Economies and Their Transformations.* Cambridge: Cambridge University Press.

Jackson, Michael. 2002. Familiar and Foreign Bodies: A Phenomenological Exploration of the Human-Technology Interface. *Journal of the Royal Anthropological Institute* (n.s.) 8 (2): 333–46.

James, Susan Donaldson. 2010. Does Dick Cheney Have a Pulse? July 15. http:// abcnews.go.com/Health/dick-cheney-heart-operation-vice-president-ready-heart/story?id=11170179#.UapvAmQbcwM (accessed June 6, 2012).

Jameson, Fredric. 2002. *A Singular Modernity: Essay on the Ontology of the Present.* London: Verso.

Jensen, Anja Maria Bornø. 2010. A Sense of Absence: The Staging of Heroic Deaths and Ongoing Lives among American Organ Donor Families. In *An Anthropology of Absence: Materialisations of Transcendence and Loss*, edited by M. Bille, T. F. Sørensen, and F. Hastrup, 68–84. Copenhagen: Springer Press.

Kantrowitz, Adrian. 1990. Origins of Intraaortic Balloon Pumping. *Annals of Thoracic Surgery* 50: 672–74.

Kleinman, Arthur. 1999. Moral Experience and Ethical Reflection: Can Ethnography Reconcile Them? A Quandary for "The New Bioethics." *Daedalus* 128 (4): 69-97.

———. 2006. *What Really Matters: Living a Moral Life Amidst Uncertainty and Danger*. Oxford: Oxford University Press.

Koechlin, Florianne. 1996. The Animal Heart of the Matter: Xenotransplantation and the Threat of New Diseases. *Ecologist* 26 (3): 93-97.

Koenig, Barbara. 1988. The Technological Imperative in Medical Practice: The Social Creation of a "Routine" Treatment. In *Biomedicine Examined*, edited by M. Lock and D. Gordon, 465-96. London: Kluwer Academic Publishers.

Kopytoff, Igor. 1986. The Cultural Biography of Things: Commoditization as Process. In *The Social Life of Things: Commodities in Cultural Perspective*, edited by A. Appadurai, 64-91. Cambridge: Cambridge University Press.

Kuhn, Thomas S. 1962. *The Structure of Scientific Revolutions*. Chicago: University of Chicago Press.

Laidlaw, James. 2002. For an Anthropology of Ethics and Freedom. *Journal of the Royal Anthropological Institute* (n.s.) 8: 311-32.

———. 2010. Agency and Responsibility: Perhaps You Can Have Too Much of a Good Thing. In *Ordinary Ethics: Anthropology, Language, and Action*, edited by M. Lambek, 143-64. New York: Fordham University Press.

Lambek, Michael. 2003. *The Weight of the Past: Living with History in Mahajanga, Madagascar*. New York: Palgrave Macmillan.

———. 2008. Value and Virtue. *Anthropological Theory* 8 (2): 133-57.

———, ed. 2010. *Ordinary Ethics: Anthropology, Language, and Action*. New York: Fordham University Press.

Latour, Bruno. 1987. *Science in Action*. Cambridge: Harvard University Press.

———. 1999a. Circulating Reference: Sampling the Soil in the Amazon Forest. In his *Pandora's Hope: Essays on the Reality of Science Studies*, 24-79. Cambridge: Harvard University Press.

———. 1999b. Give Me a Laboratory and I Will Raise the World. In *The Science Studies Reader*, edited by M. Biagioli, 258-75. New York: Routledge.

Latour, Bruno, and Steve Woolgar. 1979. *Laboratory Life: The Construction of Scientific Facts*. Thousand Oaks, Calif.: Sage.

Lavietes, Stuart. 2003. William Glenn, 88, Surgeon Who Invented Heart Procedure (obituary). *New York Times*, Mar. 17.

Law, John, ed. 1986. *Power, Action and Belief: A New Sociology of Knowledge*. London: Routledge & Kegan Paul.

———, ed. 1991. *A Sociology of Monsters: Essays on Power, Technology, and Domination*. London: Routledge & Kegan Paul.

Leach, Edmund. 1964. Anthropological Aspects of Language: Animal Categories and Verbal Abuse. In *New Directions in the Study of Language*, edited by E. H. Lenneberg, 23–64. Cambridge: MIT Press.

Lederer, Susan E. 2008. *Flesh and Blood: Organ Transplantation and Blood Transfusion in Twentieth-Century America*. Oxford: Oxford University Press.

Lévi-Strauss, Claude. 1966. *The Savage Mind*. Translated by John Weightman and Doreen Weightman. Chicago: University of Chicago Press.

———. 1969. Nature and Culture. In his *The Elementary Structures of Kinship*, 3–11. Boston: Beacon Press.

Lieberman, Daniel E., and Brian K. Hall. 2007. The Evolutionary Developmental Biology of Tinkering: An Introduction to the Challenge. In *Tinkering: The Microevolution of Development*, edited by G. Bock and J. Goode, 1–19. Chichester, U.K.: John Wiley & Sons.

Littleton, Betty L. 2004. Celebrating the History of ASAIO Smithsonian Event. *ASAIO Journal* 50 (6): lxvi–lxvii.

Livingston, Julie. 2005. *Debility and the Moral Imagination in Botswana*. Bloomington: Indiana University Press.

———. 2012. *Improvising Medicine: An African Oncology Ward in an Emerging Cancer Epidemic*. Durham: Duke University Press.

Livingston, Julie, and Jasbir Puar, eds. 2011. Interspecies (special edited collection). *Social Text* 29 (106): 3–14.

Lock, Margaret. 2002. *Twice Dead: Organ Transplants and the Reinvention of Death*. Berkeley: University of California Press.

Lowe, Celia. 2004. Making the Monkey: How the Togean Macaque Went from "New Form" to "Endemic Species" in Indonesians' Conservation Biology. *Cultural Anthropology* 19 (4): 491–516.

———. 2008. Extinction Is Forever: Temporalities of Science, Nation, and State in Indonesia. In *Timely Assets: The Politics of Resources and Their Temporalities*, edited by E. E. Ferry and M. E. Limbert, 107–28. Santa Fe: School for Advanced Research Press.

Lundin, Susanne. 1999. *The Boundless Body: Cultural Perspectives on Xenotransplantation*. Ethnos 64 (1): 5–31.

Lundin, Susanne, and Markus Idvall. 2003. Attitudes of Swedes to Marginal Donors and Xenotransplantation. *Journal of Medical Ethics* 29: 186–92.

Lyons, Dan. 2000. Diaries of Despair: The Secret History of Pig-to-Primate Organ Transplants. Report, Uncaged Campaigns. www.uncaged.co.uk/xeno.htm (accessed May 2013).

Maeder, Thomas, and Philip E. Ross. 2002. Machines for Living. *Red Herring* 113: 41–46.

Malinin, Theodore I. 1979. *Surgery and Life: The Extraordinary Career of Alexis Carrel*. New York: Harcourt Brace Jovanovich.

———. 1996. Remembering Alexis Carrel and Charles A. Lindbergh. *Texas Heart Institute Journal* 23 (1): 28–35.

Malinowski, Bronislaw. 1926. *Crime and Custom in Savage Society*. London: Kegan Paul.

———. 1922. *Argonauts of the Western Pacific*. London: Routledge and Kegan Paul.

Marks, Jonathan. 2003. 98% Chimpanzee and 35% Daffodil: The Human Genome in Evolutionary and Cultural Context. In *Genetic Nature/Culture: Anthropology and Science Beyond the Two Culture Divide*, edited by A. Goodman, D. Heath, and M. S. Lindee, 132–52. Berkeley: University of California Press.

Mattingly, Cheryl. 2010. *The Paradox of Hope: Journeys Through a Clinical Borderland*. Berkeley: University of California Press.

McLean, Sheila, and Laura Williamson. 2005. *Xenotransplantation: Law and Ethics*. Hants, U.K.: Ashgate.

———. 2007. The Demise of UKXIRA and the Regulation of Solid-Organ Xenotransplantation in the UK. *Journal of Medical Ethics* 33: 373–75.

Mead, Margaret. 1935. *Sex and Temperament in Three Primitive Societies*. New York: W. Morrow.

Men in Black. 1938. *Time*, June 13, p. 44.

Michaels, Marian. 1998. Xenozoonoses and the Xenotransplant Recipient. In *Xenotransplantation: Scientific Frontiers and Public Policy*. Annals of the NYAS, vol. 862, pp. 100–104. New York: New York Academy of Sciences.

Miéville, China. 2009. *The City & The City*. New York: Ballantine Books.

Miller, G. Wayne. 2005. *The Xeno Chronicles: Two Years on the Frontier of Medicine Inside Harvard's Transplant Research Lab*. New York: Public Affairs Press.

Mol, Annemarie. 2002. *The Body Multiple: Ontology in Medical Practice*. Durham: Duke University Press.

———. 2008. *The Logic of Care: Health and the Problem of Patient Choice*. New York: Routledge.

Mol, Annemarie, Ingunn Moser, and Jeannette Pols, eds. 2010. *Care in Practice: On Tinkering in Clinics, Homes and Farms*. Saarbrücken, Germany: Transcript-Verlag.

Montgomery, Sy. 2006. *The Good Good Pig: The Extraordinary Life of Christopher Hogwood*. New York: Ballantine Books.

Murray, Mary. 2006. Lazarus, Liminality, and Animality: Xenotransplantation, Oonosis, and the Space and Place of Humans and Animals in Late Modern Society. *Mortality* 11 (1): 45–56.

———. 2007. Xenotransplantation and the Post-human Future. In *Organ and Tissue Donation: An Evidence Base for Practice*, edited by M. Sque and S. Payne, 152–68. Maidenhead, U.K.: Open University Press.

———. 2011. Xenotransplantation, Xenozoonosis and Contemporary Imaginings of Monstrosity. *Sites* (New Zealand) 8 (1): 108–28.

NCB (Nuffield Council on Bioethics). 1996. *Animal-to-Human Transplants: The Ethics of Xenotransplantation*. London: The Nuffield Council.

New AZ Law Banks Any Moves Toward Human-Animal Hybrid. 2010. *Arizona Daily Star*, May 10.

Nicewonger, Todd. 2011. Fashioning the Moral Aesthetic: An Ethnographic Study of Antwerp Trained Fashion Designers. Ph.D. diss., Teachers College, Columbia University, New York, N.Y.

NPR (National Public Radio). 2012. Unusual and Ridiculous Stories Involving Potential Threats to Our Future. Aired Aug. 31 on *Wait Wait . . . Don't Tell Me!* http://www.npr.org/2012/09/01/160405716/the-carl-alert-system (accessed May 2013).

Ohse, C. W. 1993. Sewell's Pump. *Guthrie Journal* 63 (1).

Ong, Aihwa, and Nancy Chen, eds. 2010. *Asian Biotech: Ethics and Communities of Fate*. Durham: Duke University Press.

Ortner, Sherry. 1974. Is Female to Male as Nature Is to Culture? In *Woman, Culture and Society*, edited by M. Z. Rosaldo and L. Lamphere, 67–87. Stanford: Stanford University Press.

Page, Brian. 1997. Restructuring Pork Production, Remaking Rural Iowa. In *Globalising Food: Agrarian Questions and Global Restructuring*, edited by D. Goodman and M. Watts, 97–114. New York: Routledge.

Pálsson, Gísli. 2011. Life at the Border: Nim Chimpsky at the Nature-Society Divide. Unpublished manuscript.

Papagaroufali, Eleni. 1996. Xenotransplantation and Transgenesis: Im-moral Stories about Human-Animal Relations in the West. In *Nature and Society: Anthropological Perspectives*, edited by P. Descola and G. Pálsson, 240–55. New York: Routledge.

———. 1997. Human and Animal Gene Transfers: Images of (Non-) Integrity in Greece. In *Gene Technology and the Public: An Interdisciplinary Perspective*, edited by S. Lundin and M. Ideland, 35–47. Lund, Sweden: Nordic Academic Press.

Patience, Clive, Yasuhiro Takeuchi, and Robin A. Weiss. 1997. Infection of Human Cells by an Endogenous Retrovirus of Pigs. *Nature Medicine* 3: 282–87.

Pirsig, Robert M. 1974. *Zen and the Art of Motorcycle Maintenance: An Inquiry into Values*. New York: William Morrow and Company.

Pollack, Andrew. 2012. Move to Market Gene-Altered Pigs in Canada Is Halted. *New York Times*, Apr. 4.

Pols, Jeannette. 2012. *Caring at a Distance: On the Closeness of Technology*. Chicago: University of Chicago Press.

Pompidou, Alain. 1995. Research on the Human Genome and Patentability: The Ethical Consequences. *Journal of Medical Ethics* 21: 69–71.

Raines, Lisa J. 1991. The Mouse that Roared. In *Transgenic Animals*, edited by N. First and F. P. Haseltine, 335–46. Stoneham, Mass.: Butterworth-Heinemann.

Rice, Tom. 2003. Soundselves: An Acoustemology of Sound and Self in the Edinburgh Royal Infirmary. *Anthropology Today* 19 (4): 4–9.

Richardson, Ruth. 1996. Fearful Symmetry: Corpses for Anatomy, Organs for Transplantation? In *Organ Transplantation: Meanings and Realities*, edited by R. Fox, L. O'Connell, and S. Youngner, 66–100. Madison: University of Wisconsin Press.

Richtel, Matt, and Kevin Sack. 2012. Facebook Adds Feature for Organ Donor Status. *New York Times*, May 2, p. A14.

Robinson, Donald B. 1976. *The Miracle Finders: The Stories Behind the Most Important Breakthroughs in Modern Medicine*. New York: McKay.

Rollin, Bernard E. 1995. *The Frankenstein Syndrome: Ethical and Social Issues in the Genetic Engineering of Animals*. Cambridge: Cambridge University Press.

———. 2006. *Science and Ethics*. Cambridge: Cambridge University Press.

Rose, Nikolas. 2007. *The Politics of Life Itself: Biomedicine, Power, and Subjectivity in the Twenty-First Century*. Princeton: Princeton University Press.

Schlaudraff, Udo. 1999. Xenotransplantation: Benefits and Risks to Society (review). *Bulletin of Medical Ethics* (Mar.): 13–15.

Schrag, Zachary M. 2010. *Ethical Imperialism: Institutional Review Boards and the Social Sciences, 1965–2009*. Baltimore: Johns Hopkins University Press.

Schroeder Family and Martha Barnette. 1987. *The Bill Schroeder Story: An Artificial Heart Patient's Historic Ordeal and the Amazing Family Effort That Supported Him*. New York: William Morrow and Company.

Sharp, Lesley A. 2001. Commodified Kin: Death, Mourning, and Competing Claims on the Bodies of Organ Donors in the United States. *American Anthropologist* 103 (1): 1–21.

———. 2002a. Bodies, Boundaries, and Territorial Disputes: Investigating the Murky Realm of Scientific Authority. *Medical Anthropology* 21: 371–81.

———. 2002b. Denying Culture in the Transplant Arena: Technocratic Medicine's Myth of Democratization. *Cambridge Quarterly of Healthcare Ethics* 11 (2): 142–50.

———. 2006a. Babes and Baboons: Jesica Santillan and Experimental Pediatric Transplant Research in America. In *Beyond the Bungled Transplant: Jesica Santillan and High Tech Medicine in Cultural Perspective*, edited by K. Wailoo, P. Guarnaccia, and J. Livingston, 299–328. Chapel Hill: University of North Carolina Press.

———. 2006b. *Strange Harvest: Organ Transplants, Denatured Bodies, and the Transformed Self*. Berkeley & Los Angeles: University of California Press.

———. 2007. *Bodies, Commodities, and Biotechnologies: Death, Mourning, and Scientific Desire in the Realm of Human Organ Transfer*. New York: Columbia University Press.

———. 2009. Bioengineered Bodies and the Moral Imagination. *Lancet* 374: 970–71.

———. 2011a. Imagining Transspecies Kinship in Xenotransplantation. *Sites* (New Zealand) 8 (1): 12–39.

———. 2011b. The Invisible Woman: The Bioaesthetics of Engineered Bodies. *Body and Society* 17 (1): 1–30.

———. 2011c. Monkey Business: Interspecies Longing and Scientific Prophecy in Experimental Xenotransplantation. In Interspecies (special edited collection), edited by J. Livingston and J. Puar. *Social Text* 29 (106): 43–69.

———. 2012. Animal Familiars in Laboratory Science. Conference paper, American Ethnological Association Annual Meeting. New York, N.Y.

———. Forthcoming. Perils Before Swine: Biosecurity and Scientific Longing in Experimental Xenotransplant Research. In *Bioinsecurity and Vulnerability*, edited by N. N. Chen and L. A. Sharp. Santa Fe: School for Advanced Research Press.

Shukin, Nicole. 2009. *Animal Capital: Rendering Life in Biopolitical Times*. Minneapolis: University of Minnesota Press.

Skloot, Rebecca. 2010. *The Immortal Life of Henrietta Lacks*. New York: Crown Publishers.

Soper, Kate. 1995. *What Is Nature?* Oxford: Blackwell.

Star, Susan Leigh, and James R. Grieseman. 1999. Institutional Ecology, "Translation," and Boundary Objects; Amateurs and Professionals in Berkeley's Museum of Vertebrate Zoology, 1907–39 [originally published in 1989]. In *The Science Studies Reader*, edited by M. Biagioli, 505–24. New York: Routledge.

Stark, Laura. 2011. *Behind Closed Doors: IRBs and the Making of Ethical Research*. Chicago: Chicago University Press.

Starzl, Thomas E. 1992. *The Puzzle People: Memoirs of a Transplant Surgeon*. Pittsburgh: University of Pittsburgh Press.

Starzl, Thomas E., J. Fung, A. Tzakis, S. Todo, A. J. Demetris, I. R. Marino, H. Doyle, A. Zeevi, V. Warty, M. Michaels, et al. 1993. Baboon-to-Human Liver Transplantation. *The Lancet* 341 (8837): 65–71.

Stone, Glenn Davis. Forthcoming. Biosecurity in the Age of Genetic Engineering. In *Bioinsecurity and Vulnerability*, edited by N. N. Chen and L. A. Sharp. Santa Fe: School for Advanced Research Press.

Strathern, Marilyn. 1992. *Reproducing the Future: Anthropology, Kinship, and the New Reproductive Technologies*. New York: Routledge.

Suchman, Lucy, Randall Trigg, and Jeanette Blomberg. 2002. Working Artefacts: Ethnomethods of the Prototype. *British Journal of Sociology* 53 (2): 163–79.

Sunder Rajan, Kaushik. 2006. *Biocapital: The Constitution of Postgenomic Life*. Durham: Duke University Press.

Svendsen, Mette N., and Lene Koch. Forthcoming. The Life, Suffering and Death of the Research Piglet in Experimental Neonatal Research. *Current Anthropology*.

Sykes, Megan, Anthony d'Apice, and Mauro Sandrin. 2003. The Ethics of Xenotransplantation: Position Paper of the Ethics Committee of the International Xenotransplantation Association. *Xenotransplantation* 10: 194–203.

SyncardiaSystems, Inc. 2012. SynCardia Honored with Two Gold Stevie® Awards at the 2012 American Business Awards[SM] (Press Release, June 20, 2012). Tucson, Ariz.: Syncardia.

Sypniewski, D., G. Machnik, U. Mazurek, T. Wilczok, Z. Smorag, J. Jura, and B. Gajda. 2005. Distribution of Porcine Endogenous Retroviruses (PERVs) DNA in Organs of Domestic Pig. *Annals of Transplantation* 10 (2): 46–51.

Taussig, Karen-Sue. 2004. Bovine Abominations: Genetic Culture and Politics in the Netherlands. *Cultural Anthropology* 19 (3): 305–36.

Taylor, Janelle S. 2005. Surfacing the Body's Interior. *Annual Review of Anthropology* 34: 741–56.

———. 2011. The Moral Aesthetics of Simulated Suffering in Standardized Patient Performances. *Culture, Medicine and Psychiatry* 35 (2): 134–62.

Terrall, Mary. 1998. Heroic Narratives of Quest and Discovery. *Configurations* 6 (2): 223–42.

———. 2006. Biography as Cultural History of Science. *Isis* 97 (2): 306–13.

Turner, Victor. 1967. A Ndembu Doctor in Practice. In his *The Forest of Symbols: Aspects of Ndembu Rituals*, 359–93. Ithaca, N.Y.: Cornell University Press.

Uncaged. 2007. Victory for Uncaged Against Cruelty of Pig Organ Transplants. Dec. 9. http://www.uncaged.co.uk/news/2007/victory.htm (acessed May 2013).

VAD for Kids Is Honored. 2012. *Medical Design* (online journal), http://medicaldesign.com/prototyping/vad-kids-honored (accessed Aug. 14).

Vanderpool, Harold Y. 1999. Commentary: A Critique of Clark's Frightening Xenotransplantation Scenario. *Journal of Law, Medicine and Ethics* 27: 153–57.

van Kammen, Jessica. 2003. Who Represents the Users? Critical Encounters Between Women's Health Advocates and Scientists in Contraceptive R&D. In *How Users Matter: The Co-Construction of Users and Technologies*, edited by N. Oudshoorn and T. Pinch, 151–71. Cambridge: MIT Press.

Vesalius, Andreas. 1973. *The Illustrations from the Works of Andreas Vesalius of Brussels*. Edited and translated by J.B. de C.M. Saunders and Charles D. O'Malley. New York: Dover Publications.

Voronoff, Serge. 1925. *Rejuvenation by Grafting*. Translated by F. F. Imianitoff. New York: Adelphi.

Wainwright, Tim, and John Wynne. 2008. The Transplant Log: An Audio-Visual Diary from Harefield Hospital by Artists in Residence (book, DVD, and Web page, www.thetransplantlog.com). Edited by V. Hume. London: rb&hArts, University of the Arts, London, London College of Communications, and Arts Council, England.

Weiss, Brad. 2012. Configuring the Authentic in the Value of Real Food: Farm-to-Fork, Snout-to-Tail, and Local Food Movements. *American Ethnologist* 39 (3): 614–26.

Weiss, Robin A. 1998a. Retroviral Zoonoses. *Nature Medicine* 4: 391–92.

———. 1998b. Transgenic Pigs and Virus Adaptation. *Nature* 391: 327–28.

Willis, Paul. 2000. *The Ethnographic Imagination*. Oxford: Blackwell Publishers.

Youngner, Stuart J. 1990. Organ Retrieval: Can We Ignore the Dark Side? *Transplantation Proceedings* 22 (3): 1014–15.

Zigon, Jarrett. 2008. *Morality: An Anthropological Perspective*. Oxford: Berg.

DeVries, William, 193–194n25, 196n47
"Diaries of Despair." *See* Uncaged
Dolly the Sheep, 73, 186n32, 188n38
donors and organ donation. *See* organ
    donation; organ transfer
doxa, 30
Durkheim, Emile, 32, 33

Edel, May and Abraham, 32, 181n3
empiricism, 3–4
engineers, 15, 104–125, 190n3; genera-
    tions of, 22, 105–107, 115, 119, 190n2,
    194n29; humor, 117–118; patient
    contact, 122–123, 137–138, 177; and
    "soft" science, 120; as technicians,
    138, 142; women, 119–125
ethics: denial of, 70; ordinary, 36, 49,
    181n8. *See also* bioethics; morality;
    moral philosophy; principlism
ethnography, 7, 11–15, 16–17, 18, 30–35,
    176, 180n14, 180–181n16, 181n1,
    181n3, 183–184n12, 186n30, 196n46
ethos, 3, 11, 33, 37, 183; experimental,
    4–9, 15–24, 55, 66, 87, 150, 154,
    162
Evans-Pritchard, E. E., 33
experimental subjects. *See* patients: as
    experimental subjects
experimentation, 4, 6–7, 10; conjectural
    research, 4, 19; high-risk, 68–72

farms. *See* animals
Five Freedoms (U.K.), 71, 77, 186–187n3
Food and Drug Administration (FDA)
    (U.S.), 5, 143, 159–160, 162
Fox, Renée, 100, 102, 168
Franklin, Sarah, 47, 51, 80, 93, 161,
    180n15, 186n32, 188n38
Friedman, David, 8, 27, 67, 93–95, 103,
    110, 190nn6–7, 191nn8–9, 191n11,
    192n13
Friedman, Eli, 95–98, 192n16
Fuentes, Agustin, 62
future, imagined, 3, 10, 11, 18, 20–21,
    23–24, 27, 46, 47–48, 113–114,
    147, 151, 159–160. See also *longue
    durée*

genetically modified organisms (GMOs),
    163
genomics, 14, 52, 79, 82, 88, 147, 171–172,
    182n2, 189n49
Gluckman, Max, 33
Goodall, Jane, 61–62, 183–184n12
Green, Matthew, TAH recipient, 1–3
Guyer, Jane, 8, 11, 23–24, 27, 48, 65, 149,
    152–153

Haraway, Donna, 42, 54, 61, 87,
    183–184n12
Hardy, James, 69, 185–186n26
harm, 22
healthcare disparities, 9, 14, 17, 44–45
heart, "artificial" or mechanical, 2, 11,
    44, 94, 101, 104–119, 120–121,
    128–130; as bridge to transplant, 13;
    natal, 4, 194n30; noise, 45, 111,
    142–143, 182n12, 197n48; patients, 13,
    44, 113, 114*Fig*.11, 117*Fig*.12. *See also*
    Total Artificial Heart (TAH);
    Ventricular Assist Device (VAD)
Helmreich, Stefan, 15–18
hepatitis C, 45, 70, 189n45
heroics, 15, 45, 50, 100, 153. *See also* hope;
    hubris; scientific imaginary; virtue in
    science
historical. *See* temporality in science
Hitchcock, Claude, 69, 185–186n26
HIV/AIDS, 44–45, 70, 77
hope, 13, 39, 46–48, 77, 85, 153, 162,
    167–170; "hope technologies," 47;
    political economy or politics of, 9, 13,
    24, 25–26, 48–49; paradoxes of, 18, 29
Houghton, Peter, 133–146, 196n45, 196n47
hubris, 47, 56, 70, 152–153
human/animal divide, 55, 57–59, 87, 89,
    172. *See also* hybridity; interspeciality
hybridity, 19, 53–54, 59, 61, 67, 164, 171,
    172, 174, 178; anxieties about, 46, 69,
    83, 84–89, 151, 171–172, 197–198n6;
    embodied, 22, 42–44, 46, 50, 51, 83.
    See also interspeciality

imaginary. *See* moral imagination;
    scientific imaginary

mechanical organs. *See* heart; kidney; Total Artificial Heart (TAH); Ventricular Assist Device (VAD)

Medawar, Peter, 185n21

medical imaginary, 9, 181–182n9. *See also* moral imagination; scientific imaginary

Medicine Meets Virtual Reality (MMVR), 22

Miéville, China, 150

miraculous in science, 2. *See also* heroics; hope; hubris

Mol, Annemarie, 17, 37, 56, 176, 177, 180n13, 180n14, 197n1

monsters, 53, 61, 70, 84, 86, 88, 92, 163, 172–173, 183n10; Cheney, Dick, 111

moral imagination, 9, 25–26, 36–37, 66; in bioengineering, 90–146; moral aesthetic, 64*Fig.*3, 116–118, 127, 154; moral hierarchy, 64; paradoxes, 18, 29–30, 36, 38, 46, 107, 149–150, 167; in xeno science, 50–89, 151, 152–153. *See also* heroics; hope; hubris; visual representation

morality, 6, 29–35, 37–49, 179n6, 180n9, 180n15; biotechnologies, 29; -in-the-making, 37, 49; messiness, 16, 123; multiplicity of frameworks, 16; neutrality, 3–4, 14, 93, 143–147, 173–174; scientific, 3–9, 15–16, 18, 175; sentiment, 15–18, 22

moral philosophy, 6–7, 31–35, 37, 49, 60, 70, 180n9, 180n14, 181n3, 181n5

Murray, Mary, 86, 88

nanotechnology, 179n5

narratives, 16, 103–104, 115, 144–145, 149, 180n11, 196n46

National Health Service (NHS) (U.K.), 2, 135

National Institutes of Health (NIH) (U.S.), 160, 182n4

National Science Foundation (NSF) (U.S.), 118

nature, 54, 56–57, 57–61, 121; domesticated, 57, 58, 60, 81, 84; feral, 57–58, 79, 81, 188n43; human use of, 57;

naturalization, 56–57, 58, 65–66, 88, 174–175, 178; nature/culture divide, 57, 60; as other, 65; remaking, 55, 61; in science, 59–61, 63–66; unnatural, 58; wild, 57–58, 60, 63, 65. *See also* monster

NoXeno, 71

Nuffield Council on Bioethics (U.K.), 71, 187n34, 187n36, 188n37

objectivity, 3–4

Old Yeller, 81

Olsen, Donald, 99–100, 126, 128, 129*Fig.*14, 193n22, 193–194n25, 196n41

organ donation: brain death, 8, 13; cadaveric, 4, 13, 14, 21, 37, 139–140; as gift, 38

organ transfer (allotransplantation), 4, 12, 20–21, 29–30, 91, 172, 180n10; organ scarcity, 2, 25, 26, 48, 139–143, 149, 172, 176, 178; organ scarcity as trope, 20, 38; as reciprocity, 38; as second life and rebirth, 4, 25, 37; in U.K., 2; in U.S., 7, 37–38; waiting lists, 25

organ transplant. *See* organ transfer; transplantation

pacemaker. *See* defibulator

Pálsson, Gísli, 57, 80

Papagaroufali, Eleni, 46, 168, 182n2

patients, 13; African-American, 44–45, 69; children, 5, 15, 38, 45, 51, 69, 79, 111, 188–189n44; economic survival, 13, 25; as experimental subjects, 5, 10, 35, 174, 184n18; as "implantees," 14, 133–146; post-surgical life of, 7–8, 27–28; vulnerability, 44–45, 133–146

perfusion pump, 8, 94–95, 112, 115, 132, 191–192n11

pharma, 47, 81, 159

pigs, 3, 11, 39, 44, 50, 51, 52–53, 63–64, 64*Fig.*3, 65, 67, 74, 77, 81, 82–83, 147, 166, 183n6, 183n8, 189n46; Enviropig (Canada), 171; humanized, 43, 49, 50, 82, 86, 153–154, 159; industrial food production, 81–82, 84, 171, 177–178,